Advance Praise for *The Cancer Survivor Handbook*

"These days, more and more of us survive cancer, for longer and longer. Yet until now very little has been written to prepare people for life after treatment. Beth Leibson's wide-ranging *The Cancer Survivor Handbook* fills that gap brilliantly, with solid advice, sensitivity, and even a dash of humor."
—Elinor Nauen, health writer, former editor of special health sections for *Newsweek*

"A beautifully written book that distills the wisdom that replaces denial when cancer diagnosis strips away our delusion of invincibility. The tone will calm your anxieties as you recognize your own worried thoughts in these pages, which offer real solutions. Beth Leibson, who has been diagnosed with cancer three separate times, proves herself not just a strong writer, but a remarkably strong woman indeed."
—Kasia Moreno, editorial director, *Forbes Insights*

"This beautiful book is empathic, practical, heartbreaking, and inspiring. It's obviously essential for anyone fighting cancer or anyone who loves someone who is—but more than that, it is a memoir of survival and an introduction to many people united only by a diagnosis. Leibson is unafraid to address the questions survivors actually have (*What will happen to my sex drive? Can they fire me for having cancer?*) and to share her own achingly human story. Not just recommended reading—required reading."
—James C. Kaufman, professor of educational psychology, University of Connecticut, and Mensa Research Award winner

"As a 'fellow cancer cohort,' I loved this book. Beth's journey goes from data to stories to questions. She covers every topic imaginable and really, from sex to wellness, to what to say to people . . . she tells it like it is. The book has you laughing (and a little tearful), but keeps you totally engaged from beginning to end."
—Ann Fry, workplace cancer coach, *Huffington Post* blogger, founder of www.iamathriver.com

"Beth Leibson, who has been there (and back) herself, offers sound, practical advice that resonates with wisdom."
—Charles Salzberg, novelist, journalist, and three-time Shamus Award winner.

"Beth Leibson's book *The Cancer Survivor Handbook* should be on the must-read lists for cancer survivors, but what's less apparent, and just as important, is that it is a great book for psychotherapists, doctors, caregivers, and anyone else who has a relationship with someone who has had cancer. This well-researched, accessible book, helps us to understand that once the treatments and the doctor's visits are over, a new life begins. Ms. Leibson's writing is at once familiar and respectful of her subject, as well as her readers, and one feels as if they have an intimate understanding and appreciation for the ongoing process of life postcancer."
—Janet Zinn, psychotherapist

THE CANCER **SURVIVOR** HANDBOOK

THE CANCER **SURVIVOR** HANDBOOK

YOUR GUIDE TO BUILDING A LIFE AFTER CANCER

BETH LEIBSON

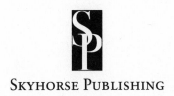

Skyhorse Publishing

Skyhorse Publishing books may be purchased in bulk at special discounts for sales promotion, corporate gifts, fund-raising, or educational purposes. Special editions can also be created to specifications. For details, contact the Special Sales Department, Skyhorse Publishing, 307 West 36th Street, 11th Floor, New York, NY 10018 or info@skyhorsepublishing.com.

Skyhorse® and Skyhorse Publishing® are registered trademarks of Skyhorse Publishing, Inc.®, a Delaware corporation.

Visit our website at www.skyhorsepublishing.com.

10 9 8 7 6 5 4 3 2 1

Library of Congress Cataloging-in-Publication Data is available on file.

ISBN: 978-1-62873-613-7

Printed in the United States of America

To Maya and Ari

CONTENTS

Introduction   *ix*

Section 1: Emotions   1

Chapter 1: Now What?   3

Chapter 2: Fear of Recurrence   23

Chapter 3: Depression and Anxiety   41

Chapter 4: Sexuality and Intimacy   65

Chapter 5: Fertility   89

Chapter 6: Other People's Reactions   111

Section 2: Career Introduction   121

Chapter 7: Returning to the Job   123

Chapter 8: Looking for a New Job   143

Chapter 9: Switching Careers   163

Chapter 10: Legal Issues   177

Section 3: Wellness Issues   199

Chapter 11: Survivorship Care Plan   201

Chapter 12: Exercise   211

Chapter 13: Nutrition   227

Chapter 14: East Asian Medicine   239

Chapter 15: Other Complementary Approaches   255

Afterword: Silver Linings, or Consolation Prizes   279

Acknowledgments   285

Appendices

   Appendix 1: Resources for Survivorship   287

   Appendix 2: Body Mass Index Table   297

   Appendix 3: A Guide to Phytochemicals   299

Index   303

Introduction

Every October, PS 3, a creative arts–oriented elementary school in New York City's Greenwich Village, holds a Halloween parade. All the children, from pre-K up through fifth grade, come to school in costume and, before their outfits get covered in paint, marker, or mud, they march around the block, led by their teachers and swarmed by adoring parents. I do mean swarmed; for a short person like me, it's important to show up early if you want a spot where your view isn't blocked.

What a view it is. Monsters and princesses, aliens and sports figures, occasional political figures, superheroes and fluffy animals. Expensive store-bought costumes as well as plenty of homemade outfits. Creativity is encouraged. One year, my son dressed up as a lump of coal, clad in gray and black with a purposefully dirty face. And then there was the year my daughter's teacher dressed as a bunch of grapes, covered head-to-toe with purple balloons; after the parade, her students had a great time popping her costume.

Afterward, there's always an assembly—a combination children's talent show, parents' band, and opportunity for the kids to model their costumes and see everyone else's outfits, now that the parents have all finished ooh-ing and aah-ing. In years past, I never stayed for the show; my curiosity was sated by the parade, and I hurried off to heed the call of my work.

But this year, my limited energy level beat out my now-less-persuasive deadlines. I'd just finished six months of chemotherapy and twenty-some sessions of radiation treatment, not to mention about a half-dozen surgeries for diagnostic purposes and to install and then remove my port (the catheter used to shoot chemotherapy treatments directly into my arteries). I was worn out, and attending the assembly would give me a chance to support my children's school, enjoy a little more cuteness, and grab a few moments of rest. At this point, I was scheduling my life around places and opportunities to sit for a bit.

So I went into the assembly and, unlike most of the parents who remained, took a seat. Actually, there weren't very many seats to take, so I ended up positioning myself on a sturdy table. Relaxing from the strenuousness of parade watching, I enjoyed the joyful noise as the kids cheered for each other, and wondered why I had always rushed off and missed this show. It was worth it just for the kids' enthusiasm and energy. Then my friend Terry came up to me and asked me, "Are you OK?" with a concerned look on her face.

"Yes, I'm fine," I said, confused. Did I look so tired? Surely people had become accustomed to *that* by now. I touched my face. It was wet; I hadn't even realized I was crying. "I'm just so glad to be here," I mumbled. I quickly left the auditorium and hurried out of the school, hoping no one else would stop me and ask questions.

According to the Institute of Medicine,[1] about half of all men and one-third of all women will develop cancer in their lifetimes. Many, of course, get cancer at very advanced years. But not everyone. Thanks to advances in detection and treatment, the number of cancer survivors in the United States has more than tripled to almost 14 million over the past thirty years. That's about 4 percent of the U.S. population. Survivors are sticking around longer, too. In the

---

1. "From Cancer Patient to Cancer Survivor: Lost in Transition," *Institute of Medicine*, November 3, 2005, http://www.iom.edu/Reports/2005/From-Cancer-Patient-to-Cancer-Survivor-Lost-in-Transition.aspx.

1970s, notes the institute, people diagnosed with cancer had a fifty-fifty shot of being alive five years post-treatment; now the figure is more like 64 percent.

The numbers of younger survivors are growing. Because we're diagnosing cancer at younger ages, and treating it more successfully, there are more and more people in the prime of their lives who've been through the cancer experience. According to the institute, more than half of survivors (59 percent) are younger than sixty-five years of age, not even old enough for Medicare. It predicts that the number of cancer survivors will hit almost 18 million by 2022, an increase of more than four million survivors in ten years.

It's a mixed blessing; I'm sorry that more and more of us are being diagnosed with cancer, but I'm glad that more and more of us are around to tell the story. At this point, cancer survivors are a sizeable alumni club. It's a club to which—fingers crossed, knock on wood—I now belong.

In other words, more and more of us have stared death in the face and lived to tell about it. Instead of closing the book on our lives, we're starting a new chapter. The challenge—and the joy—is that we have yet to write that chapter.

In a way, all that's happened to us survivors is that we no longer enjoy the illusion of immortality. No one is going to live forever, but typically people function day to day in denial. However, once someone looks at you and says, "You have cancer," that denial is gone. It's hard to plan next year's vacation or book a wedding reception venue if you think you might not be around next week. You've faced a potentially terminal disease and, after a lot of hard work, won a reprieve—but you never lose that sense that your future is uncertain, that life is uncertain.

Life after cancer often catches you off guard. At least it took *me* by surprise.

Back in 2007, about six months after I completed treatment for Hodgkin's lymphoma, I was still a mess. I was so tired that I had to rest for a half hour after taking a subway ride (even when I got a seat); I felt like I was operating at half-speed.

Lingering memory issues were still stealing my nouns; it's difficult to make a living as a writer when your vocabulary is taking a nap. My internist had just told me that my cholesterol was high and she was considering putting me on medication to treat that condition. (It went down over the year post-chemo.) Plus there were the leg pains, depression, weight gain, and oddly wavy fingernails. I'd had so many diagnostic surgeries around my neck area that I looked like the victim of an incompetent slasher. I looked in the mirror and saw a very round face with extremely short hair and no brows or lashes. I didn't recognize that lady. What was she doing in my apartment—and was she paying rent?

I was scared. Was I going to die of cancer itself? Of the cancer treatment? Or maybe of heart failure, given how hard chemo is on that precious organ and the fact that my chest received so much radiation, "the lifetime maximum," to be precise? Or maybe I'd die of a secondary cancer caused by the harsh treatment I received?

"All your symptoms are normal," my oncologist assured me. Apparently "normal" after cancer doesn't bear any relationship to "normal" under, well, normal circumstances.

"But is the cancer going to come back? I don't want to die of cancer," I worried.

"You're not going to die of this cancer," he assured me. "You've finished all the treatment, your PET scan and bloodwork look fine, you're not going to die of this cancer," he repeated. "You're going to have to get hit by a car."

Phew.

(As a side note, despite what my children would tell you, I'm much more careful crossing streets these days. I don't want to give those vehicles any encouragement. However, I still jaywalk from time to time; everyone needs a little excitement.)

Much as I appreciated my oncologist's optimism, it was still disorienting. I was done with treatment. I was starting to experience greater mobility and energy, and less pain. My hair was beginning to grow back and I'd even started menstruating again, what a thrill. Everything *should* be back to normal.

Except, of course, that it wasn't. Not quite.

This book is about my journey back from cancer. It's the book I had hoped would be out there sitting on the bookstore shelves when my oncologist told me that I'd been fine for long enough, that I probably wasn't going to die of Hodgkin's disease, that I could "go back" to life.

It also includes lots of wonderful conversations I had with amazing people, both experts and survivors—and a number of people who fit into both categories.[2] I am grateful to everyone who shared their experiences and expertise with me.

---

2. Throughout the book I refer to people who are "only" experts by their last names and survivors by their first names.

Emotions

Anyone who thinks cancer is just a physical challenge probably has never had the disease or lived with anyone who's had it. In fact, there's a good chance the person doesn't even know a cancer survivor personally.

The truth of the matter is that the diagnosis itself causes tremendous stress. One woman told me that the minute she heard the words "You have cancer," she felt as though she was surrounded by neon lights flashing "Death, death, death."

Fortunately, she's alive to tell the story, and is doing well.

Treatment brings its own set of physical, logistical, and emotional difficulties. It is frightening, it is painful in numerous ways, and it completely changes your daily life. For most people, friends and family gather around and offer support. Plus, there are usually plenty of therapists, social workers, support groups, and books to guide you through that part of the process, though it probably doesn't feel like enough to sustain you.

You don't really feel alone—or, rather, I didn't really feel alone— until after you finish treatment. The friends who visited you in the chemo suite have gone back to their lives, your schedule is so much freer, and you finally have the energy to do something.

But what is it you want or need to do?

I wasn't sure quite how to get through each day without being terrified of every twinge or sniffle. I didn't know when I'd feel confident that I was OK. I worried about some of the people I'd met: The woman in the chemo suite whose Hodgkins had come back; we chatted every session until she stopped showing up. The nice guy in the support group who left one evening and never returned. I felt sad, depressed, and anxious. And I didn't even want to consider the possibility of sharing my body with someone else when I wasn't comfortable with it myself.

People cope in different ways. Some survivors keep completely mum about their situation, while others wear their medical histories on their sleeves. Either way, though, there is much to deal with on an emotional level. This section outlines a few of those considerations.

Chapter 1

Now What?

My sixteen-year marriage ended three months before my cancer journey began. Neither experience was anything I had wanted or anticipated. I've worn glasses since I was six years old, but apparently I am near-sighted in ways beyond mere ophthalmology.

First, the kids and I adjusted to life as a threesome. Our housing had been linked to my ex-husband's job, so the three of us left the spacious, three-bedroom apartment for a cozy, four-hundred-square-foot, one-bedroom flat. (I'd been the primary caretaker, aka supplemental income, for years, so I was unsteady on my financial feet.) Fortunately, my children were young, six and ten, and didn't need a lot of space.

We learned to spread our wings. The laundry room in the basement became a permanent part of the kids' tour of our home, the twelve flights of stairs up to our apartment became our exercise gym, and Central Park, a block away, was the enormous backyard that I never had to mow. We discovered that if we crowded into the tiny bathroom and turned the light out, we got a great view of fireworks exploding in the park.

Once we'd adjusted to the spatial and financial constraints, we got our next lesson in resiliency. Two down, one to go. I was hospitalized for six days with a mystery lump in my neck that turned out to be stage-two Hodgkin's lymphoma, a type of blood cancer. I had two test-tube-sized tumors in my neck and a cantaloupe in my chest. I felt overwhelmed. I'd never had a chance to recuperate from having the rug pulled out from under me before the floor itself began to disintegrate.

But I had two young children depending on me. I didn't have the luxury of falling to pieces. So I told them, loudly and often, that I was going to be just fine. All I had to do was get through the medical treatment. They accepted that assessment immediately, and, eventually, I started to believe it myself. I hadn't realized I could be so convincing.

Friends and kind relatives appeared out of nowhere. Food arrived at my doorstep, straight from cousins Ali and James in California. Someone came to clean my apartment every other week courtesy of my sister Rachel. People accompanied me to chemotherapy, dropped off "extra food they hadn't meant to buy," handed me piles of clothing their children had outgrown, and gave me rides to radiation treatment.

The kids and I used to play a game: let's name all the people whose sofas mom has fallen asleep on. I can no longer remember exactly how many people invited us over and, as I napped, fed and entertained my children, but I am still grateful. I do remember falling asleep on the floor of the elementary school auditorium during a school-wide "festival" while children jumped in a bouncy castle, shot basketballs, and created glitter masks and spin paintings at an art table next to my snoring body. While I slept, someone made sure my children got a facsimile of lunch and enjoyed themselves. Thank you, again, whoever you are.

For months and months, I didn't think at all about reconfiguring my life. I focused on finding a good place to rest after I took the kids to school, making sure there were other adults along when we went to Coney Island or the zoo or any place where I might need to rest.

I scheduled doctor appointments when the kids were at school or made sure they had playdates planned when I had an appointment.

I figured out how much food I had to buy each day to be sure I could carry it all home and still be fully stocked. And I tried to come up with menus that hit a happy medium between Ari's preference for white food, Maya's love of hot dogs and pizza, and my fickle culinary requirements, which seemed to change every time I had chemotherapy. I realized that, as a freelancer, if I worked every day, I could squeeze in more naps than if I adhered to a traditional Monday-to-Friday schedule with weekends off. Cancer patients don't really get time off.

Denial can be a beautiful thing, and by focusing on all of these details, I was able to juggle tiny pockets of time and energy without rethinking my life goals. Managing the after-effects of divorce kept me so busy that I didn't have time to feel sorry for myself about having cancer; coping with the side effects and logistics of cancer treatment was so all-consuming that I didn't get the chance for self-pity about the divorce. I wouldn't recommend this combo meal to others, but it seems to have worked for me.

Somehow, bit by bit, tiny twist by tiny turn, I forged a new life. I'd been working as a freelance writer and editor for years, and I slowly added clients, broadening my scope from magazine articles to online publications and eventually doing some web writing and ghost writing. I started covering more health-care topics, which felt particularly compelling all of a sudden.

I took a writing class, joined a cancer support group, and made lots of new friends—people who'd only ever seen me with short, short hair. I love that they're still surprised by how long it has gotten when, really, I was only trying to get back to where I had been hair-wise as well as in other ways.

In addition, I developed stronger relationships with my children. My daughter had been very angry at first; divorce, cancer, and puberty can be a highly combustible combination. These days, we sit for hours and chat, listen to music, cook, or play cards. My son, who was so little when my life fell apart, had loved nothing more than to sit in my lap and stroke my hair, then the scarves I wore to hide my bald head, then my hair, again, when it reappeared. I've learned to allow him much more independence; he now travels around the city on his own, albeit calling in regularly so I know *where* he is being independent, with whom, and when he'll be home for dinner.

Perhaps most important, I have developed a new relationship with myself. I've learned that I am stronger than I'd ever realized, capable of trying those things that have always scared me (notably unclogging toilets and filing taxes), and much more able to ask for help when I need it. I've become fairly comfortable going places without having or being a "plus one." I've come to realize that there is life after divorce and, also, after cancer. I wonder: if I'd actually stopped to take stock of my life of my own volition, would I have been able, brave, and resourceful enough to transform my life this way?

Tracy Fitzpatrick, now a Boston-based life coach, also made changes in her life during and after her cancer diagnosis and treatment. She'd been working on a large management consulting project for the mayor of Boston when she was diagnosed. She started on the project, part-time, after her daughter was born, and had been working on it for about a year when she was diagnosed. "It was a very interesting and demanding job," she says, describing how she had enjoyed the challenge. In addition, the part-time schedule fit neatly with parenting.

After her cancer diagnosis, though, things changed for Tracy. "I realized right away that I didn't want to do that anymore." While she'd only been at that particular job for about a year, she had functioned in a similar role as consultant to nonprofit organizations and government for a number of years. The types of activities she was doing weren't exactly new to her. But, after she heard the "C" word, that sort of position just didn't feel right anymore. She didn't want to keep getting on and off of airplanes, commuting to DC and London; she wanted more control over her work schedule. Family was more important than ever.

"It also had a lot to do with the fact that I had this little girl at home, and nothing was clearer to me than that I just wanted to be with her. I wanted to be there after school and be available for school plays and that kind of stuff," says Tracy. "And I wanted to do everything I could to get healthy. That job and parenting didn't feel, at that point, like the best way to get healthy. So I did leave there, and I never looked back."

Tracy's priorities changed after cancer, and she adjusted her life to accommodate them. She did some editing to keep her hand in the working world and bring in a little cash. She realized that the important thing in her life was to see her little girl grow up. She bargained with "God or a higher power," begging, "just give me that and I won't ask for anything else. Just let me be the mother to this little girl; don't let her grow up without a mother." That was all she wanted.

"Financially, this was the craziest thing in the world for us to do, for me to leave my salary," Tracy says, pointing out that her stepson was in college at the time. "But we just made it work." Looking back on it, she's glad they could. "I feel really lucky that I had those years with my daughter." She bargained for time to focus on family and health, and got it.

When her daughter started school, though, Tracy started thinking again about her life choices. "Lo and behold, I wanted to renegotiate," she says. "It was like, well, maybe I want a little bit more."

The catch is, though, that Tracy had made this deal with herself, so she had only herself to bargain with. And Tracy proved to be a tough negotiator. "It was as if I had signed a contract, and it was being selfish and also tempting fate if I asked for more professional fulfillment or set other goals for myself," she explains. She couldn't bring herself to ask the question: "What else is there, for *me*?"

Finally, Tracy told herself, that maybe, at different points in your life, it's OK to want different things. What she wanted now was a little more than just to continue breathing. She wanted more than simply to live—she wanted to have a life.

Looking back at that immediate post-treatment period in my own life, I see that I had to sort of trick myself into finding a new life, had to make my choices and changes without being fully cognizant of what I was doing. Tracy was much more attuned to her own decisions and her own emotions. She knew what she wanted. Fortunately, we both made it happen.

The Alarm Goes Off

As it was for Tracy and me, cancer is often a wake-up call, frequently more like a loud, jolting alarm bell than a calm recitation of the daily news and weather report. It forces you to think, consciously or otherwise, systematically or not, about the life you've been leading, the choices you've made, and where you want to go from here. It's a not-so-gentle reminder that you only get so many days on this planet—and that you don't know how many you get until the countdown is over or close to it. Cancer puts you in touch with your own mortality.

Being in touch with your mortality is a powerful feeling, in good ways and bad. It can make you more appreciative of every moment in every day. In fact, many people see this as one of the "gifts of cancer." (For more on this topic, see Afterword: Silver Linings, or Consolation Prizes.)

For Lillie Shockney, director of the Breast Cancer Program at Johns Hopkins Hospital and two-time breast cancer survivor, it was more disconcerting. "I was afraid to close my eyes. I thought, 'I don't want to miss a moment of my life,'" says Lillie. "I remember thinking, 'I wonder who has stayed awake the longest in the *Guinness Book of World Records* and if they perhaps were in touch with their mortality and that's what caused it.'" Whether consciously or not, Lillie was trying to beat that world record.

"Then I also thought," says Lillie. "They were probably a manic depressive in their manic state."

Maybe, in other words, it's healthy to sit down with a friend, a good book, or an engrossing movie every now and then. Or possibly just take a nap.

In a sense, becoming aware of your mortality is really just a dose of reality. It's a reminder that we're all going to die some day. While we usually know that on some level, it's never a part of our day-to-day lives—until we feel the not-so-gentle nudge of cancer.

Tracy remembers having a "light bulb moment" when she heard a story in her support group. A single woman in the group was going through her yearlong treatment alone and had a neighbor who was very helpful to her. "She didn't know him very well, but he would go grocery shopping for her and help around the house and just be really gracious to her," Tracy explains.

Then, one meeting, the woman mentioned that her friend had had a fatal heart attack. "I remember thinking, oh my God, we all sit here thinking that 'I'm the one, I'm the one with the illness.' But he was the one who died." Tracy had assumed that she—and the other members of the support group—were in more danger of dying than the other people around them. "We think we know then what's going to happen. And we don't," says Tracy. "This division between healthy and not healthy is really just an illusion."

The reality bolt from the blue that is a cancer diagnosis often encourages people to rethink their lives. Most people do it in a more systematic way, or at least a more conscious way, than I did.

Many people, says Tracy, start out with a vague sense that they don't want to go back to their old lives, but they're not sure where they *do* want to head. There are ways to think about it systematically, by yourself or with a friend, counselor, or life coach.

Think about What Makes You Feel Alive

The first step, Tracy says, is to focus on what makes you feel most alive. As a life coach, she often has people keep track of those events, both good and bad, that elicit the strongest reaction. "It can be little things like reading an article in the newspaper or seeing a bird out the window," she says. It can be as minor as watching a group of primary school kids walk around in Halloween costumes, for instance. "Or it can be big things like a project at work or something you're doing with a child." The key, she notes, is to keep watching yourself and your reactions.

Tracy isn't referring to just the happy things in life. "You can have a real sense of engagement and a good cry at the same time," Tracy explains. "You go to a movie or you're reading a book and you're really moved by something to the point of tears," for instance. That's an indication that you are present and engaged—and that, on some level, in some way, the event is meaningful to you.

Then, as Tracy explains, you need to put a magnifying glass over those meaningful experiences and examine them closely. How did you feel about the event: positive or negative? What was it about the activity or conversation (or whatever it was) that grabbed you? Was it your role in it? Was it the environment itself? Did your strong response have anything to do with the person or people involved? It often helps, Tracy suggests, to talk with someone (like a good friend or a life coach) about these issues, or perhaps to talk in a group with other people who are also searching for meaning in their lives.

To use this approach, you need to be able to sit back and watch yourself, as though part of you is on stage and part is in the audience. For instance, Tracy says, some people come to her and say that they hate their job and never want to work in that field again. But when they analyze their responses, they realize that the job is fine—or even good in a lot of ways. In fact, they notice that about two-thirds of the time that they're annoyed at work it's because of a particular colleague or one specific aspect of the job. The aggravation caused by that nitpicking little irritant, oh, it just makes the whole work situation seem horrible. It's hard to see that in the heat of the moment. But insights like this are useful when you think about making changes.

When Miriam was diagnosed with breast cancer, she had a civil ceremony with her girlfriend of several years.

Before the diagnosis, she'd been having second thoughts about the relationship. She started seeing a therapist to talk through whether—and how—to break it off altogether. "I wasn't getting my needs met," she says. "Not that you always get your needs met in a relationship," Miriam adds. "But I just wasn't happy."

With the diagnosis, though, Miriam was worried about health insurance and, even more to the point, she didn't want to go through the treatment process alone. "I knew that if I married her, my girlfriend would stick with me and do everything she could to help me." And so would other friends. "I was scared of dying," Miriam says. So, the two of them got married.

Now that Miriam has finished cancer treatment and is fully recuperated, she's back to thinking about ending the relationship. But it's not so easy. "I'm dependent on her for health insurance now," Miriam says, with regret. At this point, Miriam can't even consider the possibility of going without health insurance which, to my Jewish mother ears, sounds wise. But there are other ways to get insurance. Being married doesn't really help Miriam feel "alive," and she is seriously reconsidering how she wants to live her life after cancer.

Visualizations can sometimes help you see things you might not think of with your "rational" mind. Tracy remembers a peak experience that she hadn't thought about in years, but popped up when she did a visualization.

"I remembered a climb I did at Yosemite, not really a climb, more of a walk, because I had a five-year-old, a niece with me." It was a family walk, with Tracy's husband, daughter, brother, and niece. "It was with family, on this beautiful, beautiful day and it was one of the first outdoor things I did after my treatment. So there I was, healthy enough to do this hike. I felt very proud of it. It was a glorious, glorious experience and I remember very explicitly feeling like it was this precious moment, and I was so grateful to be there and so happy to be there with my family and just like, this is the perfect moment."

In some ways, the experience was not so extraordinary—just a walk outdoors with a couple of family members. But, for Tracy, it summed up much of what was important to her in life. "There were elements of relationship, elements of nature, elements of gratitude, elements of physical, of feeling physically better, and elements of a spiritual connection"—all in all, sort of a shopping list of Tracy's priorities, of what she truly values. She tries to organize her life to spend more time on those elements, those experiences that bring her the most meaning.

Think about Your Accomplishments

Another suggestion Tracy makes is to think carefully about your biggest accomplishment: what made it so successful, and what made you feel so good about it? Was it the end result or the process itself? Was it the people you worked with or the type of work you did? Which of your many wonderful qualities make you most proud?

As you reflect in greater detail about your life, you will come to see some patterns, says Tracy. "What I love about my job is seeing people tapping into their own insight, their own resourcefulness, and their own wishes and yearnings and passions," she says. "As people tap into their own wisdom and their own sense of knowing themselves, they feel more forceful and confident," she explains. "They're unstoppable."

Analyzing Gives Power

Part of what was so frustrating for me, at least, about being a cancer patient was the loss of control over just about everything: my schedule, my body, my emotions, and even my cognitive functions. I couldn't eat what I used to eat, exercise the way I used to exercise, even remember phone numbers that I used to know like the back of my hand.

There were times when I lost my nouns. I don't know how many times my children wanted to know which was the "thingamajig" and which was the "whatsit." In a way, my mind was a cipher to me; no wonder they couldn't read it, either. I desperately wanted to regain some control.

Sometimes just taking the opportunity to think about what you want to do now with your "second chance at life" gives you back a sense of power over your life. "I think it is taking that step back and saying, 'OK, where have I been, and where do I think I'm going, and is this where I want to go?'" says Lillie, the breast cancer survivor who works at Johns Hopkins.

"I've seen a lot of people make very radical changes in their lives," says Tracy. For example, Lillie says she's heard of a number of "husband-ectomies" among her patients. "They'll say that though this experience isn't the cause of the divorce, they've been miserable and didn't really acknowledge how miserable they were until they went through the cancer experience," explains Lillie.

That's not to suggest that everyone changes radically. "I've also seen people go back to a very similar life but with a new attitude," says Tracy. "And they've gotten a lot more fulfillment out of their lives because of the internal shift, not because they've changed circumstances."

In my own life, I've found that it is the change in attitude that has really made a difference for me. I carry on writing and editing, I continue to hang out with my children, and I still read and walk in the park and do volunteer work and go to the theater and see friends. If you just look at my life, it seems like the only real change since cancer is that I have traded in my ringlets for straight hair— sort of the opposite of chemo curl.

But these days, I go through my routines knowing that these activities aren't things I'm stuck with. These aren't activities I do for lack of an alternative. I am living the life I want to live, the life I chose—and continue to choose.

Giving Back to Move Forward

Figuring out what I wanted to do with the rest of my life was also a matter of deciding out how to give back in some way. So many people—cancer survivors and mere mortals—helped me in so many ways through treatment and recuperation. I couldn't help them in return; by the time I was feeling physically up to it, many were no longer in my life. But I could pass it along, and help someone else. I found myself writing more and more about cancer survivorship issues—caregiving, complementary medicine, dating post-treatment, and so on. I periodically deliver food to people who are ill and homebound, and I help out at my synagogue. I'm with Matthew Zachary, brain cancer survivor and founder of the nonprofit organization Stupid Cancer, which serves young adult survivors: "You're part of the 'help to make it suck just a little bit less' community."

This work makes you feel grateful, says Elissa Bantug, a two-time breast cancer survivor who runs the cancer survivorship program at Johns Hopkins Hospital. Helping others makes you feel lucky in a way that day-to-day living doesn't always. Elissa recommends giving back to others who are going through the challenge of cancer diagnosis, treatment, and recuperation.

"I definitely think that it's very helpful to get involved in some way," says Elissa. "I think you don't realize how far you've come until you start talking to a newly diagnosed patient. Some people see it as a way to 'give back,' while others see themselves as 'paying forward.'"

Barbra is impressive in this regard. A breast cancer survivor, she's taking the training to become a Reach for Recovery volunteer and has been giving speeches for Hope Lodge, the American Cancer Society's housing program for cancer patients and their caregivers, where she stayed for much of her treatment. Barbra's also working on a fundraiser for Dana Farber Cancer Institute, where she received her care.

Beth (not me) has also become a serious volunteer. She also battled breast cancer. These days, she volunteers regularly at You Can Thrive, a nonprofit organization that offers support services for breast cancer survivors. In addition, she is very active on Internet chat rooms, answering questions and helping people feel less alone as they go through their cancer journeys. "I found that people helped me, and even if it was just people on the Internet in chat rooms and stuff," she says, "so I should help other people." Online and by phone, Beth is endlessly patient and willing to spend time answering questions and providing reassurance.

Joe, an almost-two-decade survivor of non-Hodgkin's lymphoma, didn't start out as an avid volunteer. A year after Joe finished treatment, the National Cancer Institute asked him to come back and speak to the patients on the pediatric floor, where he received treatment. "I tried, but I couldn't do it," Joe remembers. "I had this tremendous, tremendous survivor's guilt, and I couldn't look at these kids and speak to them. I just felt bad—I felt bad that they were going through what they were going through," he says. "And, honestly, I didn't know if they would make it."

"Then a good friend of mine from high school, Ryan, was diagnosed with non-Hodgkins lymphoma," Joe remembers. When Ryan died, Joe was at his wake, and he spoke. "I said this is kind of a wake-up call to me that I need to get off my ass and do something to make a difference." And so he began. "In 2002, I did a hundred-mile bike ride around Lake Tahoe with Team in Training," he says. "I like to call that my 'coming out party.'"

These days, Joe is firmly ensconced in the cancer community and volunteers at Imerman Angels, LiveStrong, Movember, and the Leukemia and Lymphoma Society. In addition, Joe marches on DC every year with One Voice Against Cancer, a collaboration of national nonprofits that appeals to the White House and Congress annually. "I try to do my part to make a difference in people's lives," he explains.

Rachel, who has survived stage-three breast cancer, is very involved with a couple of breast cancer organizations, including Living Beyond Breast Cancer and the Susan G. Komen Foundation. She does photo shoots, comments on websites, does the Komen Foundation three-day walk annually, and is a co-chair on a committee to help Komen reach out to younger women. "I think in a selfish way it makes me feel a little bit better about things," she says. "I'm actually doing something about cancer rather than just having had it happen to me. It gives me purpose."

Khit has been involved with volunteer work since she was a child. When she was growing up, her father was very involved with the PLO (Palestinian Liberation Organization). "He was friends with Yasser Arafat, and he always hosted benefits for children or families that were affected by all the Israeli and Palestinian conflict back home," in the Middle East, says Khit. Her family spent every summer in Jerusalem. "My mom would always make us take our food to people who were refugees that lived in tents."

So Khit comes by her volunteer activities naturally. These days, she puts in eighty-plus hours a week, mostly working in recruitment marketing and outreach for Imerman Angels. She's always "on." She does a lot of public speaking and organizing, and even when she's bartending, to pay the bills, she raises money for Imerman Angels. She even works when she's working out. "I've recruited about 170 of the 230 athletes that we have now at the gym," she says.

Khit loves to teach people how to work with nonprofit advocacy organizations. "I really believe that if everyone in this world could find something that they're passionate about, people in general would be better." Khit is certainly doing her part.

She also runs in marathons regularly to raise money for Imerman Angels. "I'm not running marathons because I want to show off," she says. "I'm doing it because I can, because I have the freedom to do it. I have my legs, I have the freedom to do what I want to do," she says. "In the end, I want to be remembered as someone who tried to make a difference."

Many cancer survivors become active in their communities, says Tracy, and often within the world of cancer. "A lot of people want to give something to somebody else," says Tracy. "Either they start volunteering at a wellness program or a cancer support program or they start doing fundraising or they get involved in their temple or their church communities more or they start working with kids in their volunteer time." Some people even switch their careers to something in the cancer world. (For more about career changes, see Chapter 8: Switching Careers.)

"I need to make it a meaningful aspect of my life to use it to help other people," says Mindy Greenstein, PhD, psycho-oncologist, writer, and two-time breast cancer survivor. "People did that for me." It's a way to feel good about your life, to know you did something useful with your life and with your "second chance."

Of course, helping patients isn't for everyone, Elissa warns. For some people, this sort of activity enables people to see how far they've come. For others, though, it is a crystal ball into an uncertain future and just raises the anxiety level. In her job, Elissa explains, she carefully picks whom she shares that particular piece of advice with. So before you commit to weekly sessions for a year, test it out to see whether helping others is good for your own psyche. If you're hysterical, you're no help to anyone else.

Finding Meaning through Spirituality

Volunteering isn't the only way people find meaning. As soon as Roberta was diagnosed with breast cancer, at age forty-one, she felt a change. "I became more spiritual because I felt that bad things were going to happen in my life but that God was sending me a signal that he would provide some support for me." Her feeling of being emotionally buttressed was fortunate because it was 1985, when there was much less public awareness of cancer and less support for survivors.

Roberta had always expressed herself through her body. She was a dancer until "a terrible thing happened" and she switched her priority to self-defense and she took up karate. She was very involved in politics and "and karate seemed like a practical way to protect myself during civil disobedience," she says. Under the name Florence Flowerpot, Roberta opened a karate school for women, one of the first in the city, in the late 1960s.

Two weeks before she was diagnosed with cancer, Roberta "fell in love with yoga" at Kripalu Center for Yoga and Health, a retreat center in the Berkshires. She also became friends with a woman who had had a mastectomy, the first person she met who she knew had had breast cancer. "I knew that yoga and my new friend would be my main supports while I was dealing with cancer," says Roberta.

"Karate didn't seem to honor where my energy was anymore," says Roberta. "I was very excited to be doing yoga. It really got me through the whole experience. Through yoga, through listening to tapes, through meditation." The drive toward physical self-empowerment has been replaced by a need for self-healing. Roberta started teaching yoga. "I realized that's what I wanted to do, that it was what really honored my energy."

When we think about life-threatening diseases and spirituality, people's immediate thought is about the end of life. We think about organ donation. We picture, perhaps, the priest who comes to the hospital bedside to take the terminal patient's last confession. But spirituality, especially when defined more broadly than formal religion, can provide meaning to anyone's life—even someone who intends to continue to have one.

It's not always easy to define spirituality, though most people can recognize it when they see, or feel, it. For some people, spirituality enables you to connect to other people; sometimes, it helps you find the best in yourself. Often, it is connected to our physical and emotional life. It can provide a sense of peace, purpose, and connection, says Hannah H. Gibson-Moore, LMSW, emotional support counselor at the Livestrong Foundation.

Roberta found her sense of spirituality through connection with others and meditation. Other people, notes the Mayo Clinic,[1] find it through quiet reflection in nature, laughter, singing, yoga, prayer, affirmations, journaling, or even in church, synagogue, mosque, or other formalized religious institutions. While there aren't any research studies linking spirituality to health, it is widely believed to contribute to quality of life.

Watch out for Internal Critics

With all the changes that cancer and cancer treatment bring, your ego can take a real blow. I've found I often lack the confidence I used to have. There's something about having your body fail you that jolts you out of complacency.

Since I finished cancer treatment, I find myself reading my work over and over, even more than before. I sit there revising, reading it out loud, then editing some more. I show it to one writer friend, then to another. Then I show the piece to someone who doesn't write for a living because "you are the real audience." Then I go back to the computer for one last round of editing.

This approach is not necessarily inappropriate. It's often useful to check over your work. Sometimes a little more reading over could stand me in good stead. One time, I handed in a magazine article where I typed "fat ass" instead of "fat mass." Fortunately I have an

---

1. Sheryl M. Ness, "Connecting to your inner spirit helps with cancer diagnosis," *Living with cancer blog*, November 17, 2012, http://www.mayoclinic.com/health/beliefs-and-cancer/MY02301.

editor who is highly skilled (she caught the typo) and very kind (she laughed and told me I had made her day). Then, a few weeks later, she assigned me another piece. Thank goodness.

Still, there is a line between careful editing and neurotic obsession. My typo notwithstanding, I find myself straddling—and crossing—that line more often since cancer. (Incidentally, I hate to read my work once it's in print; *that's* when I find all the ways I could have made my prose clearer, more helpful, or more interesting.)

Tracy calls these tendencies to second-guess your work "gremlins." The road to your dreams is guarded by these critics, says Tracy, these monsters and gremlins. "They would much rather have us stay safe and miserable than take a risk and go for a big dream," she explains. Logically, it seems like passion and desire should be enough to keep you on track to try something new. But unfortunately, passion and desire are no defense against the bouts of inconfidence and fear that seem inevitable. Once you've had cancer and lost faith in your body's imperviousness, it's even harder to take a chance. You worry that you aren't thinking as clearly as you were, that your reflexes aren't what they had been, and that you lack the energy you used to have. The gremlins gain ground.

The trick to eluding those gremlins, suggests Tracy, is to maintain the ability to look at yourself from afar, and to analyze your actions in an objective way. "Our critics just want to keep us small," says Tracy. "We have to learn when to listen to them—and when it is time to trust our gut and take the brave step of sending our work out into the world."

Tracy suggests paying attention to when your assessment is reasonable and when you're being just a tad (or two) too careful. The best defense against gremlins is constant vigilance. After a while, when you re-prove your own strength to yourself, the strength that has been apparent to others all along, those gremlins will recede into the shadows. Unfortunately they never really recede completely. They're always there, waiting to pounce, so you have to be on the watch all the time. Don't let them win.

Sometimes it is easier just to keep bumbling through life, rather than stop and reassess. It takes time and energy to rethink your life. Cancer just won't let you get away with continuing the status quo. As I worked through cancer treatment and single parenthood, I felt like I was just muddling along trying to get my kids to school and keep a roof over our heads. Cancer showed me—as it shows most people—that we're stronger than we'd realized. We can take that determination that we put into fighting the evil C and devote it to staring down our gremlins and figuring out our "new" lives.

Don't let those gremlins fool you. Think about what gives your life meaning, what feels like an accomplishment, and what makes you feel truly alive. Often, the answers to those questions will help you figure out what you want to do with your "second chance," despite what your anxieties hint at. You may need to talk it over, to analyze it with a friend, therapist, or support group. You'll almost certainly have to fight those gremlins along the way. Remember, though, that if you can fight cancer, you can fight a gremlin or two.

You may decide that you're happy with your life, with your friends, your family, and your career. That doesn't mean you've missed the "lesson of cancer." It just means that you figured out you've been leading the life you want all along. Realizing *that* may lead to a greater sense of appreciation.

When you think, "Now what?" you can take this chance to improve your life. Think about what makes you feel alive, about what skills and accomplishments feel like positive contributions, and about how you can find meaning in your "second chance." You'll need to learn to trust yourself (and ignore those gremlins). Ultimately, your "new life" can only lead to great things if you let it.

Frequently Asked Questions

Q: Is it normal to think about changing my life after cancer?

A: Many people see cancer as a wake-up call, an opportunity to rethink the choices they've made, the lives they've chosen, or the lives they've fallen into.

Q: What if I don't know what I want to do?

A: There are lots of ways to figure out what is meaningful to you. You can work with a life coach or a friend, or in a support group of some sort. You can analyze what makes you feel most alive and take a good look at your accomplishments.

Q: What if I don't want to change my career, but I still want to give back?

A: Many people find that volunteer work is a good way to help other people while continuing with their already established careers.

Q: If I feel good about my family, friends, and career, have I missed the "lesson of cancer"?

A: There's no overarching "lesson" for every cancer survivor. It sounds like you just figured out you've been leading the life you wanted all along. When you see that, you may well gain a greater sense of appreciation for your family, friends, and career. That's the lesson for *you*.

Q: I can see what changes I'd like to make in my life, but I feel incapable—maybe even unworthy—of seeking more. After all, I'm lucky just to be alive. Shouldn't I just be satisfied with what I have?

A: Most people have demons inside them that keep them from making changes. It is important to be aware of this—and not to give in to those instincts. You've been given the gift of life—it's your responsibility to make the most of it. Don't let the demons win.

Chapter 2

Fear of Recurrence

Soon after I finished treatment for Hodgkin's Disease, a cancer of the lymph nodes, and was declared cancer free, my neck started to hurt. Not my throat, which I could have written off as a cold, allergies, or at worst, strep—but my neck. More concerning, it hurt in exactly the same spot where I found the lump that had started me on my cancer journey.

The journey had involved three surgeries to diagnose and six months of chemotherapy, followed by twenty-four sessions of radiation to eradicate. Or at least to make it so that PET (positron emission tomography) scans came up clean. "No cancer as far as we can tell," is what they told me.

On that day, though, not only did my neck hurt; I started to feel nauseated, sweaty, and just a little woozy. I knew it was a recurrence. It had to be. What else would cause that specific type of pain in that precise location? I walked over to the bookcase and picked up the sole photograph I have of myself during chemotherapy, my face rounder than usual thanks to steroids, my naked skull wrapped tightly in a rose-colored scarf, my brow- and lash-less eyes hidden by my glasses.

I keep this photo around to remind me of how far I've come. It's sort of a visual way to maintain my perspective. I hadn't meant for it to show me the path I might walk down again. I tried to hold the hand-made wooden frame carefully, but somehow it broke just a little bit.

I know that no one can guarantee my cancer won't come back. I am well aware that despite the heavy-duty warfare inflicted on my body, one or two itty bitty cancer cells could easily remain hidden in some obscure corner of my body. In addition, I remember that the very definition cancer is cells gone wild—those cells multiply faster than bunny rabbits, and are nowhere near as cute. My oncologist thought I was OK, but even he couldn't *really* be sure. No one could.

I realized I couldn't just stand there, holding a broken picture frame and worrying. I had to have it checked out. I was shaking as I sat down at the computer to send an email to my wonderful oncologist. I knew he couldn't schedule a scan right away, I wrote, but could I at least set up an office visit for an examination? I remember trying hard to stay calm, though now that I look back at that note, I see that I wrote "I'm a little nervous" twice in a two-and-a-half-line message.

Fortunately, my oncologist is a patient soul. Not only did he respond to my email that same afternoon; two days later, I was sitting in his office as he palpated the spot and said I was fine. The next scheduled PET scan indicated, likewise, that I was fine. I started to breathe again.

At the post-scan appointment, I asked my oncologist if my response had been normal. I asked if every cancer survivor got "a little nervous" sometimes. He said that my reaction was perfectly reasonable— "as long as you don't do this every week," and he leaned to give me the usual hug; he claims these aren't check-ups so much as "visits."

My oncologist wasn't just being nice. "Fear of recurrence is probably the number-one side effect, if you will, of the patient experience," says Elissa Bantug, a two-time breast cancer survivor who runs the cancer survivorship program at Johns Hopkins Hospital.

Technically, recurrence is the reappearance of cancer after everyone thought it was gone. It can pop up in the original spot, near that spot, or even in some other part of the body. Cancer isn't fussy. "I see fear of recurrence almost across the board, with almost every single patient," says Elissa.

Her observations are accurate nationwide; the American Cancer Society has found that 70 percent of cancer patients worry about recurrence at about one year after diagnosis. Of course, there's no guarantee that passing your first cancerversary will eliminate the worry. Every survivor I know worries about it, no matter how many times they've been told they are cancer-free.

Cancer Is Different from Other Diseases

In our society, the word "cancer" has become a metaphor for evil. Racism is a cancer, as is hatred in general. If you look at the headlines, it's almost a cliché: Republicanism is a cancer, liberalism is a cancer, homosexuality is a cancer, homophobia is a cancer. No one ever says that so-and-so is like a diabetes on the world or a multiple sclerosis on society. There's a special stigma associated with cancer.

Mindy Greenstein, PhD, psycho-oncologist, writer, and two-time breast cancer survivor, agrees. She points out that while heart disease feels like "a problem with the plumbing," cancer feels like "a malevolent force with a personality."

Cancer is considered a particularly tough disease to treat, so we don't mince words when we talk about it. We describe it, and its treatment, with war metaphors. You *fight* the disease using *weapons* such as chemo and surgery, led by an *army* of doctors. When you're finished, you've *defeated* it and you're a *survivor*. Not only is cancer a battle; our bodies are the battlefield. As Mindy explains, "When you are the battlefield, it doesn't matter who the good guys are and who the bad guys are. All the bombs are falling on you."

Cancer robs you of a sense of security in your own health. I will never again assume that I will be healthy and energetic until otherwise notified. I've been put on permanent notice. Phrases like "no pain, no gain" and "walk it off" don't mean quite the same thing anymore. There's really no way around it: cancer has played a powerful role in my life, and that part of my story will never go away. The AMBER alert will be in effect as long as I am.

That being said, there are ways to cope with the very natural fear of recurrence. The first step is to notice when the fear arises.

When You Feel It in Your Toes

All sorts of things bring to mind fear of recurrence. Medical symptoms—aches and pains that aren't easily explained and sometimes even ones that are—can set off alarm bells. As Donna, a breast cancer survivor, asks, "When is a headache just a headache?"

Elissa has had some experience with this sort of worry. After treatment, she had twelve recurrent strep infections in nine months and finally elected to do the tonsillectomy that her doctors had been recommending for years. She'd been experiencing these strep infections long before she had cancer, and they were totally unrelated to anything oncological. "It just has to do with how my body is built," she says.

"I didn't want to do it because the surgery is awful in adults." It is especially difficult for someone with her history of strep infections and her consequent scar tissue in the back of her throat. Elissa decided, though, that it was finally time to stop proctrastinating and have the surgery.

Before she went under the knife, Elissa had asked her mother to bring her laptop to the hospital after the surgery. "She looked at me like I was crazy," Elissa remembers, but her mom didn't ask questions and dutifully followed Elissa's request. "The first thing I did when I woke up from surgery was to log on to see if the pathology report from the tonsils had come back," Elissa admits.

She'd experienced no warning signs of throat or topical cancer. It wasn't as though her cancer treatment had been the previous week; at this point, Elissa was about a decade out from her initial breast cancer diagnosis. But even in her morphine-influenced state, cancer was what Elissa thought of, the first thing she wanted to check, even though she knew there was no scientific reason to worry and no rational explanation for her concern. "I don't know of a single case study of breast cancer ever traveling to the tonsils. It doesn't really go there," says Elissa who works in the cancer field and knows what she's talking about. "Topical cancer is very rare as a primary cancer." All of that information didn't come into play. Elissa was still worried about the possibility of the Big C.

Tito, a fellow Hodgkin's survivor, had a similar experience. His tumor was in the neck. When he felt a tightness in his throat one day, more than a decade after he finished treatment for cancer, he thought immediately about his lymph nodes. Were they OK? Was this a recurrence? Tito made an appointment to see his oncologist.

While he was waiting to see his doctor, Tito hit the Internet. "Google is your worst enemy," he says. "You put in anything, it relates back to cancer." He wasn't finding anything reassuring. Fortunately, he tore himself away from the computer long enough to see the doctor, who diagnosed a completely treatable case of esophagitis. (He's fine.)

When It Starts

For some people, fear of recurrence starts the minute they finish treatment. After all, during treatment, you are busy, busy, busy doing everything in your power to fight the cancer. You have an array of oncologists, surgeons, radiologists, nurses, and technicians leading the way. You have almost daily interactions with pills and needles, radiation, and surgical knives.

Then, suddenly, it's over. "See you in six months," my oncologist said. In an instant, I went from fighting full throttle to trying to remember my kids' spring school vacation schedule so I could schedule a follow-up appointment. I went from doing everything I possibly could to, well, doing not much of anything at all.

As I stood there making the follow-up appointment with my oncologist's secretary, I remembered a woman in my support group who started worrying about staving off cancer as soon as she finished treatment. She begged her oncologist for one more dose of chemo, just for good luck. He smiled, she told us, and said no.

At the time, I thought she was nuts. I was more like Elissa. She could have been telling my story when she described how she "went through treatment like a kid, marking the days off on the calendar. Like you would for the last day of school." I, too, couldn't wait to walk out the door after my twelfth session of chemotherapy.

Cancer would be over, I thought, as soon as treatment was. I never, ever wanted to see that oncology suite or radiation treatment waiting room again. I shared that sentiment with my favorite oncology nurse, and she just smiled. I guess people in the oncology field are accustomed to patients being anxious to escape their office.

It turns out that the specter of cancer doesn't part ways when you shake your oncologist's congratulatory hand. "Some of the hardest times I ever had were after treatment was over," says Elissa. "Living with this fear, dealing with this fear of what I had just gone through and the fear of what was going to come next."

Fear kept Elissa up almost every night for a year and a half. "I was doing self-breast exams in the shower all the time. And when I say all the time, I mean every single day," she explains. "I feel robbed of peace of mind. Cancer has taken that from me, and it will never come back."

As I stood there scheduling my follow-up appointment, I understood how the woman in my support group had felt. I too wished there was some action I could take to know for sure that there were no cancer cells lurking in my body. I realized that I'd never get to cross cancer off the list of my life.

Medical Appointments Are Scary

It's not just aches and pains that remind survivors of cancer. When I look at my calendar and see that I have an appointment for a scan, blood work, or a check-up, I get nervous. I realize that these things are all meant to reassure me. The results will show that I'm fine. Or, at worst, they'll find a speck of cancer so infinitesimal that a wave of the magic oncology wand will eradicate it.

Somehow, though, it always feels like a reality check. I'm walking through life feeling as though I'm in good health. Then one of those appointments pops up on my calendar and all of a sudden my body starts acting weirdly. Something starts to hurt, I feel a little lethargic, or there's some generalized ache or pain.

I used to go back to the cancer center for tests or exams every two or three months for Hodgkin's Disease, and then it slowed down to every six months. That's pretty standard, according to the National Cancer Institute (NCI). People usually go back every three to four months during the first few years after treatment and then once or twice a year after that, notes the institute. Some of these appointments are just physical examinations and check-ins; other times, survivors may have to submit to blood work, imaging (such as mammograms or sonograms, PET scans, or CT scans), or other tests.

Even when they become less frequent, though, onco appointments still cause all sorts of bells to go off. "I get very nervous before any screening or surveillance test," says Elissa.

Even non-cancer-related appointments can remind us of our mortality. Rochelle, survivor of a rare soft tissue cancer, tries to avoid all medical appointments, even a dozen years after finishing her cancer treatment. "I can't stand going to the doctor, so my first thought is always let me see if I can *not* go," she says. "I often feel anxious around medical appointments of any kind, like appointments that other people wouldn't give a thought to."

"I burned my thumb last year. It was a very bad burn," she remembers. But Rochelle didn't want to step inside a doctor's office, even for something that clearly had nothing to do with oncology. Doctor's offices spook Rochelle these days. "I just looked online for what you should do for a very bad burn," she says. She followed the instructions carefully, but her thumb still blistered severely. In the end, Rochelle ended up having to go to the doctor anyway to have it treated, but her discomfort with any sort of medical attention made her put it off until absolutely necessary. Most of us survivors can relate—anything to avoid triggering the paranoia that so often accompanies medical appointments post—cancer treatment.

Other Scary Things

Beyond twinges and appointments, some people have other little quirks that lead to stomach butterflies and dizziness. Any little reminder can prove worrisome. Elissa found, for instance, that she felt it in the pit of her stomach while she was being handed a pink Race for the Cure T-shirt by a Susan G. Komen Foundation representative. She was doing a good deed, making a positive contribution, but still it made her just a little ill.

Because you can't always predict when these "little reminders" will trip up your day, it helps to have a few tools to deal with the fear. While you may always be briefly stupefied by a reminder of cancer, you needn't be completely immobilized.

Time Is a Tool that Heals Wounds

It's a cliché, but there's some truth to it, at least in this context. Time really is an effective healer for the fear of cancer recurrence. It helps to be kind to yourself, to give yourself some time to mourn what you lost, and prepare to move on.

As Elissa reminds her patients, "Recuperating from cancer is a marathon, not a sprint. You're going to have good days and bad days, good hours and bad hours, and you have to be patient with yourself." For most patients, she explains, it gets better over time, though time in this sense is measured more in months than in days or weeks. Elissa counsels patience to her patients. "We took part of your life," she tells them. "But we plan to give you back many more years."

Of course, she admits that it's easier to say that to someone else than it is to accept it for yourself. "It took me a year to get my body back after cancer treatment," says Elissa. "It took me two years to kind of get my emotions and my spirit around this idea of embracing cancer," meaning dealing with the disease.

I know that this is true for me. I no longer wake up in the morning surprised to be doing so. I can have a stuffy nose without worrying about nasal cancer (does that exist?). I can go to the ophthalmologist without worrying about eye cancer (is there such a thing?). I can even walk past—and into—the medical facility that saved my life without feeling my stomach churn and scanning the room for the nearest toilet or trash can.

Life is easier when you can become comfortable with that uncertainty. It's not easy. Often, that level of comfort comes as time passes.

The Tool of Seeking Support

I can attest that it also helps to know you're not alone in your fears and concerns.

I was lucky to find a post-treatment support group. From what I understand, there aren't a lot of those around; often, support programs focus on people going through treatment. If you're "cancer-free as far as we know," the thinking goes, you don't have emotional issues, either.

I was able, though, to find a group where I could kvetch to people who understood what I was experiencing. I got to go every month to a room full of people who knew that I might not be rational for feeling nauseated a block away from my hospital, for instance, but that I wasn't crazy. I got to talk with a bunch of (mostly) women who knew all the right questions to ask, the appropriate times and ways to be reassuring, and when to just let me be. I got to hear other people's stories and know I am not alone. I also got the chance to share my hard-earned knowledge and understanding. After all, no one understands cancer survival like someone who's been there.

If the group isn't going to meet soon when I start to worry about recurrence, I've found that the best thing I can do is to call up a friend who's had cancer. People who haven't experienced cancer firsthand tend to try to be a Pollyanna when I want to kvetch or offer advice when I just want someone to listen. It's hard for them to predict the most helpful response. Fellow cancer survivors are more likely to understand what type of support I need.

Tracy Fitzpatrick, life coach and cancer survivor, once told me that we survivors have "a PhD in cancer," and while I certainly didn't apply for the degree (and would like a refund on my tuition), I have to agree. We survivors have all learned something along the way. There's nothing like sharing bald heads to bond a friendship—though I don't recommend taking a razor to your skull in your quest to find a fellow traveler.

In her professional capacity, Elissa concurs. "I definitely recommend talking to other people to normalize the behavior, whether it's a support group or one-on-one or an online community." It is important, she says, for survivors to "know that they're not alone and that other people are experiencing the same things."

A Nod to Caregivers

Elissa points out an interesting side note to this fear of recurrence. Survivors, like me, often forget about those kind, caring, and often-underrated caregivers, the loved ones who are around us every day as we go through treatment and recuperation.

"In some ways, I think being a caregiver is a lot harder than being the patient," says Elissa. "The patient kind of gets a pass to behave badly or to say you don't want to deal with anybody right now." Caregivers get no such sympathy.

In fact, because caregivers lack that not-so-enviable experience, they often don't really understand the thread of irrational thoughts and fears that race through a cancer patient or survivor's brain. "They can empathize but they don't really know," says Elissa.

Most survivors have their ups and downs. "There were some times when I would say, 'Why can everyone pretend that cancer didn't happen?'" Elissa remembers. "Then I would say, 'Why doesn't anybody ask me how I'm feeling? Do they think that I'm not going to be OK?' In a sense, there's no way to win," says Elissa. It's a very tough job with really long hours and lousy pay.

Caregiver preservation is just one more reason to turn to a fellow survivor when you need an ear.

The Tool of Knowing When to Worry

A little knowledge can also help stave off the fear of recurrence. I have learned to stop and think before I push the panic button. If I can remember bashing my skin into a friend's coffee table, chances are those leg pains aren't related to cancer. If I tried a new exercise routine the other day, I can take those muscle aches as an indication of increasing strength, not growing tumors.

On those days when I can't locate a bruise or remember an explanation, though, it can take some deep breathing—and sometimes an email or two—to consider the possibility that I'm not dying. I'm lucky that my oncologist and friends are generally available and always kind.

It helps to remember that not everything is a sign of cancer. The American Cancer Society lists the following as warranting discussion with your health-care provider:

- Return of the cancer symptoms you had before (such as a lump or a new growth where the cancer first started)

- New or unusual pain that seems unrelated to an injury and does not go away
- Weight loss without trying
- Bleeding or unexplained bruising
- A rash or allergic reaction, such as swelling, severe itching, or wheezing
- Chills or fevers
- Unusual headaches
- Shortness of breath
- Bloody stools or blood in your urine
- Lumps, bumps, or swelling
- Nausea, vomiting, diarrhea, loss of appetite, or trouble swallowing
- A cough that doesn't go away

Just because the American Cancer Society recommends talking with your health-care provider, though, doesn't mean that you need a full-body scan and seventy-five blood tests every few weeks. Sometimes getting something checked out can just mean talking with your health-care provider, describing your symptoms, and having the worrisome spot examined and palpated.

Since my medical oncologist uses email, I get swift responses to little questions, plus easy prescription refills. Equally important, he lets me know quickly when I need to make an appointment to go into the office. He gently reassures me while keeping my hypochondriacal tendencies in check.

Elissa, too, walks that fine line—on both sides. "I think it's really important for patients to trust their intuition and their bodies," she says, noting that she typically gets four or five angst-ridden phone calls a week. By the same token, "it's really easy to open up Pandora's box and start having tests looking for cancer." Patients can end up with unneeded radiation and stress as little nothings have to get checked out. Not to mention the physical discomfort and scheduling challenges of fitting all those tests and follow-up appointments onto a full calendar.

Instead, Elissa typically starts by talking with her nervous patients. "I talk to patients about very tangible things: about what to look for, what are signs of recurrence." We have to remember that, unfair as it is, we can still get the same colds, infections, arthritis, and heart problems that hit people who haven't had cancer. Germs don't know that we've already been through the medical wringer. They show no compassion.

When the Nightmare Happens

Hodgkin's disease wasn't my only time at the circus. A few years after I finished treatment, at just about the time when my check-ups were becoming less frequent, one of those "now that you're forty" routine mammograms turned up cancer in my right breast. The good news was that it wasn't a recurrence; it was a new primary cancer. (The fact that it was another "new" cancer, not a recurrence or metastasis of the Hodgkin's lymphoma, meant that my prognosis was much better than it would have been otherwise.) It was a little baby primary, too. It didn't seem fair, though. I'd already done the whole cancer thing.

Besides, I'd always thought my breasts were my friends. They held up my bathing suits, fed both my children when they were infants, and were, somehow, completely symmetrical. When it turned out they were harboring fugitive cancer cells, though, our peaceful relationship changed. The ensuing lumpectomy also changed their symmetry, so despite my breast surgeon's meticulous work and miniscule scar, things no longer look exactly the same, even when I'm dressed. For the first time in my life, my breasts looked slightly different, like most women's breasts do naturally. They looked different, and I felt different; in that sense, we were a matched set.

My calendar started filling back up again with mammograms, sonograms, MRIs, blood work, and check-ups with my breast surgeon as well as my medical oncologist. I collect MDs like some people collect comic books. Unfortunately, though, I can't fold them into plastic bags, stow them in the closet, and forget about them until I'm in the mood.

When I finished treatment for the breast cancer, I went to my internist and told her, "Check everything. I want to make sure there's no cancer in my fingernails or anywhere else."

I scheduled as many doctor appointments as I could. Alas, as often as I have asked, they still haven't created one of those metal-detector-style sensors that can locate rogue cancer cells anywhere in the body. But according to the docs, my colon, eyeballs, teeth, and lymph nodes were all certifiably healthy. My blood and urine were normal, and there were no signs of Hodgkin's. My breasts passed inspection; that cancer was at bay, too. Knock on wood.

I was done with cancer, I'd moved on. I'd even started writing a book about "life after cancer."

Then, two years after the first one, while I was working on this very book, those evil cells popped up in my left breast. A slightly abnormal MRI followed by a looks-OK-to-me mammo. I convinced myself that it was just too early for me to have cancer again. Surely I was entitled to a couple of years off for good behavior.

A biopsy confirmed the unhappy story. I had my third primary cancer; I'm lucky that I haven't had an actual recurrence. I've come to realize that life after cancer means not only fear of recurrence, but also the very real possibility of an actual recurrence or, in my case, a new cancer. (Or, more precisely, two new cancers. But who's counting?)

I've also learned that getting another cancer, which I had thought was my worst nightmare, isn't actually the end of the world. As I faced my second breast cancer diagnosis, I took a couple of long, solitary walks in Central Park and decided to chop off both breasts. It would mean no more mammograms and no more breast cancer. (I know that it doesn't mean no more cancer altogether; I'm optimistic, not completely delusional.) Now, one double mastectomy and reconstruction later and here I am, still finishing up that book on life after cancer. Determined to live that life after cancer.

Elissa had a similar experience. When her greatest fear came to fruition—when she had a recurrence of breast cancer (an actual recurrence, not a second primary)—Elissa was terrified. Her doctors recommended a mastectomy, not a lumpectomy as she had the first time. Just get rid of the whole breast, they suggested.

That approach, intense as it was, didn't seem sufficient for Elissa. "I opted to do a bilateral mastectomy because of the fear of recurrence. I just felt like I was living under this dark cloud, I was so terrified that my cancer was going to come back," Elissa says. "I felt like cancer had already taken so much of my life away from me and it had already monopolized three years of my life. I couldn't live under that black cloud anymore." Now, breast cancer is no longer an option for Elissa.

We have both faced down our worst nightmares and are both still here to tell the story.

Gaining Perspective

One of the gifts of the passage of time is gaining perspective. I've realized, for instance, that as a single mom and freelance writer, I only have so much time and energy to devote to fretting. I need to target my efforts more effectively. In other words, I must stop worrying so much about cancer and focus on getting my daughter into college and preparing my son for high school. (In New York City, getting into high school is almost as arduous as applying to colleges, except there's less travel.)

Elissa agrees. "You can point out that if someone spends a lot of time worrying about cancer that either they won't have cancer—in which case they've spent a lot of time worrying for no reason—or they will have cancer—and they still wasted all that time," she says.

It's not so easy to just tell someone to stop worrying, as you've probably observed on issues unrelated to cancer. It simply doesn't work; most people don't have an on-off button for worrying. Saying "don't worry" is sort of like saying "don't think about a pink elephant."

"It's a matter of finding the right way to do it, finding something that works in your life, a way that is culturally sensitive and meaningful," Elissa explains. That's why it can be helpful to have a friend, relative, or counselor—whether online, in a group, or in person—who understands what you're feeling and can provide the support you need.

Ironically, my second cancer—in my left breast—was discovered on a routine mammogram. No pain, no lump, not even a tiny little twinge of paranoia. I'd been worrying about my neck but hadn't had a second thought about my breasts. I'd been wasting my time with misguided worry. (The other breast cancer, not surprisingly, was a little less unexpected.)

It helps that I know, for the most part, when I'm going to fret. Weird aches and pains, scheduled medical appointments, and my own personal bugaboos give me the heads-up. I now recognize these feelings as just that: concerns, not diagnoses. When I worry—and I do, though much less often than I used to—I call a sympathetic friend, check in with my oncologist, and remind myself that the scares outweigh the diagnoses.

On a bad day, I try all three.

Frequently Asked Questions

Q: Do other people worry about recurrence? Or am I the only one?

A: Almost all cancer survivors worry that their cancer will come back. It is possibly the most common "side effect" of the disease.

Q: What kinds of things will make me more nervous?

A: Every survivor has his or her own triggers. Typically, people worry when they feel an odd ache or pain, something they cannot attribute to a recent accident or illness. Often, doctor's appointments, too, start people worrying about recurrence. In addition, there are those individual little reminders that vary from person to person. It helps to try to figure out what your triggers are; then you can try to anticipate them.

Q: What can I do to be less worried?

A: The cliché says that time heals all wounds. I'm not sure it completely alleviates all concerns, but it certainly does help with fear of cancer recurrence. The more you see other medical things happen, for instance, the more you realize that not every ache is cancer. It could, for instance, be just a touch of arthritis.

Q: What if I actually do get another cancer, or a recurrence?

A: You've already proven that you can beat cancer. This time, you'll know more going into it. You know how cancer works and what diagnosis and treatment are like. You've got doctors you trust and friends you can count on. If—God forbid—you are diagnosed with another cancer, you'll just get another chance to prove your strength and resilience.

Chapter 3

Depression and Anxiety

For Mindy, the hardest part of cancer hit after treatment was over. When she was first diagnosed with breast cancer, she felt anxious for a few weeks, but then she got caught up in intricacies of decision making and the logistics of juggling treatment, work, and home life. She was too industrious to feel anxious. "I felt like I was actively mobilized against the invader; I had something concrete to keep me busy," she explains

Once treatment was over, though, it was a different story. "After I had my final surgery for my implants, I was really depressed for a couple of weeks," she remembers. "The hardest moment for me was the recognition that, shit, I have to go back to just living a life again. Somebody had taken me to the abyss, showed me the bottom, then brought me back," she remembers. "Now I'm just supposed to live? Not live in fear," she clarifies. "But just *live*."

"While I was in treatment, I was active," says Mindy. "But the 'after' part is a much more passive experience," she adds. "I have all this knowledge that I wish I never had. Now I have to just live my life. In some ways, that knowledge can make your life better," says Mindy. It adds to your appreciation of the small things, for starters. Tracy talks about how she used to hate taking her daughter to the mall—until after cancer. Now she's grateful for any time spent together.

But enhanced appreciation isn't always the case, says Mindy. "In other ways, it's like this boulder that sits on your shoulder," a weight that can feel like too much to bear.

Matthew, who was diagnosed with brain cancer when he was a senior in college, was also very dejected by the diagnosis. He was a pianist and composer who had several CDs to his name already, at the tender age of twenty-one. He was ready to head out to California to attend graduate school. "I don't drink, and I don't smoke, and I don't do drugs. But the fact that I had no pre-existing vices was not in my favor." He would have liked a way to distract himself, to escape the reality of the disease, even temporarily. Not, I'd like to point out, that he advocates alcoholism or drug addiction as a helpful response to a cancer diagnosis.

His left hand had lost its ability to perform fine motor skills; in fact, it was this symptom that led to the discovery of his disease. "I couldn't arpeggiate. I could only play a single note at a time," Matthew remembers. His doctors told him that he'd never play piano again. That assessment turned Matthew's entire existence upside down. He had to change all his plans. He didn't go to grad school, and, after he graduated from college, he moved back in with his parents. He was depressed and not sure what to do with himself. But he kept at the piano. "I just started playing, just sat down at the piano," he remembers. Five years later, his hand was retrained, and Matthew could play as he had before.

As soon as he was able, Matthew put out a new CD, though by this point, he'd gotten a job in marketing and advertising, so music was more of a hobby than a profession for the now-twenty-six-year-old. "I developed a bit of a reputation as the kid with brain cancer who was told he'd never play piano again." Soon enough, his reputation spread, and Matthew started getting gigs playing piano for cancer patients. Performing really helped pull Matthew out of his funk.

Anxiety comes in different forms for different people. I found, for several years, that my nemesis was geography. There were specific places that, without fail, made me jittery and nauseous.

I received my cancer treatment in a facility in lower Manhattan. The facility was fine—clean and welcoming and (this is important during chemo) without a whiff of any possibly objectionable smell. The nurses were friendly, the patients were kind, or asleep, and my oncologist always dropped by with a word of encouragement. He occasionally brought a gift. My children still snuggle under a soft red afghan emblazoned with the words "Lilly Pharmaceutical— making chemistry personal."

I really did appreciate the many kindnesses I experienced from my health-care professionals during treatment. Perhaps I didn't appreciate them sufficiently to actually calm down when I was there. While I was in cancer treatment, I was thoroughly terrified of the building, and I had to give myself a pep talk every time I crossed the threshold into the chemo suite. I often went with a friend, Claire, and she had to literally give me a gentle push each time into the room for treatment.

The oncology nurses were wonderful; they had obviously seen this before. The first thing they did once I got situated in my chair was to inject anti-anxiety medication directly into my port. Within a few minutes, with the happy drugs coursing through my veins, I was calm. They could do the blood work necessary to find out if my white and red blood cells were healthy enough to withstand the chemotherapy that would then drip into me for several hours.

For about two years after I finished treatment, I couldn't walk in that area without experiencing a little inexplicable nausea. When I say "that area," I'm not talking about the chemo suite itself or even the medical center building. I mean the entire three-block radius around that caring, life-saving facility. There's a large and lovely bookstore in the area that I couldn't even walk into without feeling sick.

Even when I took my kids there to pick out books, I experienced equal parts maternal love and pride at my little readers and anxiety and queasiness at the location. I have no idea how my body distinguished between those nausea-inducing shelves of books and stores in other neighborhoods that had no effect whatsoever on my insides.

Over time, I calmed down and found I could not only walk around the area but even enter the medical center without my heartbeat quickening. I don't remember a specific moment when I realized that stepping on those linoleum squares didn't affect my well-being. It was more of a gradual acceptance and calming.

Then a long-time friend was diagnosed with breast cancer. I recommended my oncologist, and my friend took me up on the suggestion. I was glad. I wanted her to be OK, and the best way I could think of to help was to share the name of the man who saved my life.

Somehow, though, it didn't register that seeing my oncologist would mean she'd be going to the same physical office and, worse yet, the same chemo suite where I had been treated. I wanted to be a good, supportive friend and visit during her treatment, and, in fact, I went to almost every one of my friend's chemo sessions. But she probably had no idea how difficult that was. I believe in facing your fears, but it's not exactly something I looked forward to.

Visiting with my friend during the three or four hours she was receiving the chemotherapy drip meant walking over the threshold and staying in that room without a drop of pharmaceutical encouragement. I hadn't realized that I'd been classically conditioned, like Pavlov's dogs. I saw that room and wanted to vomit.

My favorite oncology nurse was still working in the suite when I went to see my friend. After we chatted for a few moments catching up, with her admiring my hair, I asked her for some anti-anxiety medication. Just a little bit, for old times' sake, I said. She seemed to think I was joking.

I realized that I needed to do something about this neighborhood-a-phobia. By going back over and over, and having nothing traumatic happen to me while I was there, I was able to conquer the fear and reclaim the neighborhood. I can even go to the bookstore now, as our bookshelves will attest.

Seizing the Day

Lillie Shockney, RN, BS, MAS, professor and administrative director of the Johns Hopkins Cancer Survivorship Program, has a different emotional response to her breast cancer. She finds herself, even years after her cancer experience, unable to stop and smell the roses. "I'm still in that mode of watching the sun come up and saying, I don't want to miss a moment of my life," she says. "So I'm trying to cram even more into my days than is probably realistic and I've been that way for a long, long, long, time."

Part of it has to do with her childhood. The day she turned six years old, Lillie's father took her out to the cow barn and told her, "You will now do the work." He said, "You and your brother will be out here milking cows twice a day before school and after school, and you'll be on the tractor on the weekends." So, at an age when most girls are focusing on conquering the alphabet and hopscotch, Lillie became accustomed to putting in a fourteen-hour work day. "Play time was not part of that day," she says. "I was taught that productivity is incredibly important and you must accomplish, accomplish, accomplish."

Fast forward a number of years, and Lillie is still putting in fourteen hours a day at her job at Johns Hopkins. At the same time, she's busy taking care of her family and dealing with her own two diagnoses of breast cancer. Instead of trying to make more time for herself, Lille focuses on increasing her work time to sixteen or eighteen hours a day.

Recently, Lillie learned that she has a heart condition that could be very serious. Her primary care doctor wants her to slow down. "I told her that I don't know how to," Lillie says. "I feel guilty when I'm less productive. People say to me, 'Gee, you do the work of three people,'" Lillie explains. "Well, I think I'm supposed to. I wonder, why isn't everyone else doing that?" Her need to contribute became only stronger after her cancer diagnosis, as she wanted to do as much as she could as quickly as possible. She knows she needs to try to slow down, but she just isn't sure how.

All Too Common

Cancer survivors face a variety of emotional challenges: stress, anxiety, depression, you name it. They can range from depression to workaholism and from anxiety to a fear of a particular geographic area and can interfere with a survivor's lifestyle and relationships. Sometimes it is hard to distinguish which is depression and which is anxiety, but in the end, it all just gets in the way of getting on with your life.

Prepare yourself; here comes a statistical interlude: According to MD Anderson Cancer Center, about 70 percent of cancer survivors experience emotional difficulties. In fact, according to researchers at UCLA, the prevalence of depression among survivors is three to five times greater than in the general population. Research at the Livestrong Foundation suggests that 51 percent of cancer survivors experience depression or sadness. The bottom line is that it's rough to be a cancer survivor—and studies prove it.[1]

As many as half of all cancer survivors have some symptoms—anxiety, depression, fatigue, cognitive dysfunction—after treatment,

---

1.   "How Cancer has Affected Post-Treatment Survivors: A Livestrong Report," *The Livestrong Foundation*, June 2010, https://assets-livestrong-org.s3.amazonaws.com/media/site_proxy/data/56bb2f9bd97d32e96194e3c62b6ee97e84a4726b.pdf.

according to Andrew Miller, MD, professor of psychiatry and behavioral sciences and director of psychiatric oncology at the Emory University Winship Cancer Institute. "If you really talked to cancer patients," says Miller, "you'd be hard-pressed to find anyone not affected in some way." (Sexual dysfunction is also sadly common. If this is part of your life, just hold on for a few more pages; we deal with that in the next chapter.)

The bottom line is this: Finishing with cancer treatment doesn't mean finishing with cancer's emotional toll. It is not at all unusual to experience some sort of stress, anxiety, or depression. In fact, sometimes the stress increases when treatment is over.

It's hard to know when to worry about your symptoms. According to the Dana Farber Cancer Institute,[2] if you have any of the following signs for more than two weeks, you should probably talk to your doctor:

- Feel worried, anxious, sad, or depressed
- Have emotional numbness
- Feel overwhelmed, out of control, shaky
- Have a sense of guilt or worthlessness
- Feel helplessness or hopelessness
- Display irritability and moodiness
- Have difficulties concentrating, feel "scatterbrained"
- Cry a lot
- Focus on worries or problems
- Become unable to enjoy things like food, sex, or socializing
- Avoid situations or things that you know are really harmless
- Have suicidal thoughts

---

2. "Your Emotions After Treatment," *Dana Farber Cancer Institute*, accessed December 2, 2013, http://www.dana-farber.org/For-Adult-Cancer-Survivors/Caring-For-Yourself-After-Cancer/Your-Emotions-After-Treatment.aspx.

There are also some body changes that suggest anxiety or depression, according to Dana Farber:

- Weight gain or loss that you can't explain
- Insomnia or increased need for sleep
- Racing heart
- Dry mouth
- Increased perspiration
- Upset stomach
- Diarrhea
- Headaches, aches, and pains

Everybody copes with these emotional challenges in his or her own way. After all, the person you were before cancer is the same person you are after it. If you tend to be shy and nervous before diagnosis, you won't be transformed into a loudmouth the minute you walk out of your last treatment. If you tend to be a glass-half-empty kind of person before diagnosis, you probably won't become a Pollyanna after treatment. As much as you may be affected by cancer, it doesn't alter your basic make-up.

"A life with cancer is just like a life without cancer," says Mindy, wearing her onco-psychologist hat. "Except that everything is magnified."

There are many ways to cope with life after cancer. It helps to understand your own coping techniques.

Coping Techniques: Superstition

In the back of my underwear drawer, where some women hide jewelry or money or stash their most risque lingerie, I have three purple hospital gowns. Purple, incidentally, is my favorite color. The items are made of soft flannel, covered with delicate flowers and butterflies, relatively attractive for hospital gowns—and never worn.

My oldest friend, who lives more than one thousand miles away and wanted to be present in my life as I went through cancer, made these for me when I was diagnosed with Hodgkin's disease. They arrived a few days after I got out of a six-day stay in the hospital. I wasn't an inpatient again with Hodgkin's, so I didn't use them as I went through treatment for that part of my cancer journey. It never occurred to me to don hospital gowns, even ones with purple flowers, at home. I stuck them in the back of my bureau.

Friends suggested that I donate the hospital gowns to a cancer organization, or at least give them to someone who was facing a hospital stay and might be able to put the gowns to good use. I worried, though, that if I gave them away, I'd be demonstrating an inappropriate level of arrogance. *Here you go, universe, I won't ever need these items again, so I can bestow them on someone else.* I didn't want to dare the universe to prove me wrong, to provide me with an opportunity to put these hospital gowns to good use. So the three purple flannel gowns stayed in my underwear drawer, serving a weirdly magical, somehow prophylactic purpose.

Then I had breast cancer and was treated with an outpatient lumpectomy. No overnights in the hospital, no need to wear a hospital gown. The ones I owned stayed stashed away and forgotten.

The second time I was diagnosed with breast cancer, I had a double mastectomy and reconstruction. I knew it would be a big surgery and was told I'd probably be on the OR table for about ten hours. (It was twelve.) I was also told I would be in the hospital for three to five days. My surgeons eventually split the difference and released me after four.

When I packed my bag to take to the hospital, I put in clean clothing to come home in, toiletries, the almighty insurance card, my cell phone, and a few books in case I had enough energy to read. I wasn't sure what I'd be in the mood for, having never selected post-operative reading material before. Besides, I figured I wasn't going to be the one carrying the bag home. (Thanks again, Deni.) But I didn't bring the purple hospital gowns. It might have been a subconscious decision, but my conscious mind had honestly forgotten all about them.

Mindy had a similar experience with a wig. When she was facing chemotherapy for breast cancer, she was told she would probably lose her hair. She was worried that a bald psychologist wouldn't look professional, so she had a wig custom made. When it was done, it sat at the wigmaker's shop, waiting for Mindy to pick it up, which she decided she would do as soon as she needed to wear it. She did pay for the wig, of course.

Mindy never lost all her hair. It just thinned. "I just looked like someone with very unattractive, thin hair," says Mindy. Because she was never bald, she never needed the wig.

So the wig sat at the wigmaker's shop. "I didn't want to pick it up until I needed to," she says. "Then my chemo ended, and I had never picked up the wig." She'd already paid for it, but wasn't sure what to do. "I was very superstitious about what to do about the wig. Should I have it? Would that mean that I'm inviting chemo again, that I'm ready for another chemo?" she asked. "If I give it away, am I being arrogant?"

Mindy is not usually superstitious. In general, the psycho-oncologist approaches life and its challenges with great pragmatism. She calls herself "a major realist who had whole databases of my chances and my side effects and all sorts of things." Even her mantra, the phrase that helped her keep calm throughout the toughest parts of treatment, exemplifies acceptance: "You get what you get and that's what you get."

But somehow her knowledge-seeking, reality-accepting approach didn't translate into the wig situation.

"I never did anything about it," Mindy remembers. "I never even called the woman who made it. I was paralyzed about what to do because I really thought I should donate it to somebody, but I couldn't bring myself even to do that."

Mindy's wig superstition, like my own strange ideas about the purple hospital gowns, didn't hurt anyone. They didn't particularly help anyone else—notably people who could have used the attractive headpiece or the comfy hospital attire—but the superstitions worked for both of us, particularly because we were prepared to accept the consequences of our actions, illogical as we knew them to be.

Research suggests that Mindy and I aren't alone in our quirks. Studies have shown, says Stuart Vyse, PhD, professor of psychology at Connecticut College and author of *Believing in Magic: The Psychology of Superstition,* that when people imagine a particular scenario, they think it is more likely to occur. If I see myself in those hospital gowns, if Mindy pictures herself wearing that wig, we're more likely to end up there.

Is this true even if you're aware of what you're doing? Even if you know your behavior isn't logical, that it's based on an illusion?

Yes, says Vyse. "There is a growing sense that we are more than one creature in the same skin in that we have an intellect but we also have an emotional side and an intuitive side," the psychologist explains. It's not just cancer survivors, either. "I've had studies of people who were superstitious and they will say, I know this is silly, I know this can't be the case, but I'm going to do it anyway because, one, it makes me feel better and also, two, I don't want to take the chance that if I hadn't done this, things would have turned out better." So we can set out to fool ourselves, we know we're trying to fool ourselves—and it still works; it still provides reassurance.

Well, then, now that I have some empirical evidence backing up my superstitions, I'll be hanging onto those hospital gowns for a while.

Rochelle, a survivor of a rare soft tissue cancer, had a different kind of superstition? "I stuck with a job that was literally making me ill," she remembers. She'd been working in that after-school program for more than two decades, and had enjoyed it, but recent changes in the parent board created a toxic environment. "They made my life miserable," she says.

She felt like she couldn't move on. "I felt like damaged goods," she says. "How could I start something new when I had this thing hanging over my head?" says Rochelle. She felt as though looking for a new job would be tempting fate, displaying overconfidence in her health.

Not only did Rochelle feel like damaged goods because of the cancer, but she was scared of change in general. "Change has always been scary for me." Cancer made that worse. "I feel like it puts you a little bit separate from the world. It's harder to be like everybody else," says Rochelle. "I feel like other people are more carefree."

Eventually, Rochelle got up the nerve to switch jobs. "But I stayed for seven years after I finished treatment," she remembers. "The last three years were increasingly difficult."

At first glance, this seems like an example of when superstition didn't serve someone well. But given Rochelle's fear of change, her superstition about staying at her job makes a lot of sense. Finding and starting a new job ranks pretty high as stressors go. Who wants to start a new position, with all the challenges of sussing out different procedures, office politics, and even where they keep the printer paper, while it feels like the Sword of Damocles is hanging over your head? Better the "Devil wears Prada" you know than the one you haven't met yet. As Vyse suggests, if you think something may help you, there may well be a positive placebo effect; that action may, indeed, ameliorate the situation.

Vyse explains that there's pretty good evidence that if you believe in luck in a situation where you actually have to perform an action, that belief can help you. It can, as Vyse says, "actually have a positive effect on your performance." The effect is psychological, though, not magical, the psychologist adds. "If we then stamp out the belief in magic," Vyse asks, "will we be robbing people of something that would in fact objectively help them perform better?"

In short, Vyse is no high priest of rationality. "I would suggest that there are benefits to believing in superstition under certain circumstances," he says. "They're not the benefits that the believer thinks they are," he explains. "But there are psychological benefits to them."

Psycho-oncologist Mindy agrees. "It's not for me or anybody else to say whether she was making the right or wrong choice," she says. "There's no way of knowing." In the end, though, a superstition is working for you if it helps keep you calm and focused and if it helps keep that anxiety, fear, and depression at bay. If you feel better with those gowns in your drawer, then what the hey?

Vyse agrees. "As a scientist or just a human being, I know that that's the case. In other words, the alternative would be to try, because I have this view that this person is under the spell of a false belief, I would try to kick that belief out from under them and I feel like that would be a victory for rationalism and science, but the person would be left damaged by that, in terms of their ability to cope with the world." And, he wonders, how exactly would that help?

The Connecticut College psychologist talks about Pascal's Wager. "This is an old idea that is sort of a calculus about believing in God," he explains. "Heaven and the afterlife are such an enormous potential reward [for a religious Christian] that the cost of believing in God and living a Christian life seems small in relation to what you would get for it." And if it turns out that there's no heaven, well, not much was lost. The concept, developed by the seventeenth-century French philosopher, mathematician, and physicist Blaise Pascal, may have started as a theological argument, but it has evolved into a psychological one in our twenty-first-century world.

To bring the concept down from the theoretical, Pascal's Wager points out that it's no big deal for me to hold onto the hospital gowns. My apartment is small, true. But it's not *so* small that a few pieces of fabric are going to overwhelm us. In Mindy's situation, she isn't even filling up an iota of space in her apartment (though we don't know what the wigmaker is thinking). As far as we can tell, there's no real cost to hold onto these things. If by not doing anything I can avoid taking the chance that I will feel a horrible regret, well, I'm OK with that. So, it would appear, is Mindy.

Vyse offers another explanation that has to do with passive versus deliberate actions. "If you take an action and it comes out badly, there's a greater sense of regret, often, than if you fail to take an action and something bad happens," the psychologist says. It's not logical; it's purely emotional. "In other words, if you play it safe and things turn out badly, you don't feel quite as bad as if you had changed your job or if you had gotten rid of the gowns or the wig." It's all sort of magical thinking, he adds.

One possible downside to magical thinking, though, is that it could potentially be a constraining way to live. If, for instance, you need to wear your special socks when you go in for chemo in order to ensure that your platelet levels are sufficient to receive treatment then, well, you might have to think carefully about when you do your laundry. Similarly, someone who worries about having a doctor's appointment on a Friday the 13th may have to do some fancy footwork if that's the only day a specific specialist is available.

Again, though, this may not seem like a very high price tag if the benefit is big enough. Doing laundry regularly, for instance, isn't such a bad thing.

Another possible downside to this approach to magical thinking could be self-blame, says Vyse. "If you buy into the idea that your actions can affect the course of your disease, then it injects a sense of responsibility that may or may not be there," he explains.

So, let's say that I give away my purple hospital gowns, Mindy donates her wig to an alopecia organization, or Rochelle looks for a new job. Then, if any of us were to get cancer again, we might feel that we'd brought it on ourselves. "This is unfair and may actually create a sense of responsibility that is unjustified," says Vyse. Unfortunately, though, that doesn't keep people from feeling that way.

One additional concern has to do with obsessive-compulsive disorder (OCD). Someone with OCD uses a rather extreme version of magical thinking to get through the day. They might, for instance, need to wash their hands until they're scrubbed raw or need to check the that the stove is turned off so many times that it's hard to leave the apartment after dinner.

But the chasm between the sorts of superstitions we've been discussing and a medical disorder is pretty wide. "It is the case that people who have OCD often do have some rituals that are superstition oriented," Vyse says. "But the great majority of people, and children, who have such things do not go on to develop OCD."

Coping Technique: Attitude

When it comes to labeling that cup of H_2O, I tend to be a little indecisive. If I'm looking for a parking spot, applying for a job, or wondering whether I really should have brought that umbrella, I'm more of a glass-half-empty sort of person. But when it comes to things like, oh, surviving cancer, somehow my glass is half full. I never promised consistency.

I suspect my optimism has much to do with taking care of my kids. I grew up in a household built on the unsteady bricks of family secrets, so when I was diagnosed, I told my kids exactly what was going on and what the treatment would (I thought) be like. I did put a positive spin on the facts, though, telling them that I just had to do chemotherapy and radiation and then I would be fine. Cancer free. "It's just a matter of getting through the treatment," I explained. I left no room for doubt and to this day, they don't know what all the fuss was about. After repeating that often enough, I started to believe it.

There's definitely something to be said for having an upbeat attitude. We live in a society that glorifies looking on the bright side, seeking the silver lining, taking a positive attitude. Whether you put your faith in God, science, or your doctors, people want to believe they're going to be OK. Our language is littered with expressions like "life is a bowl of cherries," "there are no problems, only opportunities," and "make lemonade out of lemons." Apparently fruit is a particularly optimistic food group.

Some people claim that having a positive attitude will cure you, change your life, and maybe even make you rich. The term "positive thinking" has been a part of the American vernacular at least since Norman Vincent Peale first published the book *The Power of Positive Thinking* back in 1952. That advice certainly worked for Bobby McFerrin, an accomplished vocalist who made his name in 1988 with a song titled "Don't Worry, Be Happy."

According to the Mayo Clinic,[3] there are, indeed, certain health benefits credited to positive thinking:

- Increased life span
- Lower rates of depression
- Lower levels of distress
- Greater resistance to the common cold
- Better psychological and physical well-being
- Reduced risk of death from cardiovascular disease
- Better coping skills during hardships and times of stress

Even if you're typically a glass-half-full kind of a person, though, you don't have to maintain that approach all the time. Optimism is an attitude, not a requirement. Allow yourself to feel sad sometimes. Bottling up the sadness and anger doesn't get rid of it. I've found that the occasional good cry can lead to a lot more smiles later on.

Sometimes, interestingly, having a positive attitude can result in negative feelings. By saying that a positive attitude will solve problems, such as cure cancer or prevent recurrence, you're implying that lacking a positive attitude can cause those problems. Someone with a "bad attitude" can "bring it on themselves." Or it can lead to self-delusion; lying to yourself about your diagnosis or prognosis doesn't

---

3. "Positive thinking: Reduce stress by eliminating negative self-talk," *The Mayo Clinic*, accessed December 2, 2013, http://www.mayoclinic.com/health/positive-thinking/SR00009.

help anyone. It's especially a problem if holding that positive attitude prevents you from following the recommended course of treatment.

On the other end of the continuum from 100 percent optimists are people like Mindy. "We are absolute realists—we pride ourselves on knowing everything and not sugar-coating it, and preparing for the worst. I'm sort of the poster child for that group," she says.

Taking a realistic attitude can allow you to set appropriate goals, which may make it easier to meet those goals. But it, too, can backfire. If, for instance, you are convinced you should be 100 percent recuperated from surgery within two months but then find yourself still achy and tired at ten weeks out, you might feel like a failure.

On the other hand, if you give yourself three months, and maybe a little leeway with that, perhaps you would be able to focus on getting better rather than berating yourself. "Hope for the best, prepare for the worst" is the operative cliché here.

Barbara Ehrenreich has said, in an interview with the *Boston Globe*, "So yes, sometimes it's irritating to be around somebody who doesn't say every idea you have is brilliant, who says instead, I have these doubts," she said. "But I want to be with the person who has the doubts."[4]

Mindy talks about a variation on the theme, an approach that has been termed "defensive pessimism." That's when people are planners to the nth degree, she explains. They think of all the possible bad outcomes and come up with Plan B, Plan C, and Plan D. "Then they can put those plans in a box and relax," says Mindy. They know the plans are available if the need should arise. "But if you take that away, if you try to get them to just be optimistic and not think about the bad things, that actually makes it more difficult," she explains.

---

4. Jenna Russell, "Enough with the Bright Side," *Boston Globe*, October 11, 2009, www.boston.com/bostonglobe/ideas/articles/2009/10/11/enough_with_the_bright_side/.

While it can be helpful to think positively, it's probably more trouble than it's worth if the approach is not in your nature. It's not fair to add the burden of having to stay positive to a cancer survivor, of having to change your mind-set. Allow yourself, or other survivors, to be true to yourself. A positive outlook won't affect cancer, but it may make it easier to handle some of the challenges, logistical or emotional, that come along with survivorship. An upbeat outlook will do the trick only if it comes naturally to you. Some things you just can't fake. Especially to yourself.

Pick a Style, Any Style

The truth is, though, that most of us are somewhere in the middle of that continuum. We're not complete optimists, but we're not total rationalists, either. Sometimes we even move around between the two philosophies, like I do when I am more confident in my ability to fight cancer than to find a parking spot on a busy city street.

"There's no right or wrong," says Mindy. "Most of us are really on the continuum somewhere in between," she adds. "Problems arise when you have two different people with two different styles at opposite ends." Perhaps most important, it arises when the two people don't respect each other's philosophy. "The realists often don't respect the deniers; they feel like they're not processing the stuff that they need to process," says Mindy. "And the deniers feel like realists are too negative."

Again, we are the same people after cancer treatment that we were before diagnosis. "You learn who you are over time," says Mindy. "By the time you've had cancer, you've probably had other crises in your life, and you come to learn how you've dealt with things in the past," she adds. While occasionally some people find that cancer is a game changer, most deal with the disease and its aftermath with their familiar style.

"I think that for the most part, our coping styles are fairly constant," says Mindy. "If you're a positive thinker during treatment, you were probably that way beforehand, and it will be what comes most naturally to you."

Some people change their approach day to day. Someone might be in denial most of the time, but then become realistic at one point, or vice versa. Mindy, for instance, reacted one way the first time she was diagnosed with breast cancer, but had a completely different style when the cancer recurred.

"When I had my original diagnosis, I researched everything," she says. "I already knew more than I wanted to because of my work, but on the other hand, I hadn't worked with a lot of breast cancer patients, so there was plenty for me to learn."

But when the cancer came back? "The second time around, I wanted to know as little as possible," says Mindy. That confused some people who remembered her research frenzy, but it worked for Mindy. She dealt with the recurrence and moved on with her life.

"Research is not on your side that being positive is the best way of coping with it for everybody," she says. Optimism isn't necessarily better than realism. The biggest challenge is when people don't accept the way you deal. "The problem occurs when I want to impose my style on someone or that person wants to impose her style on me," Mindy points out. In our culture, Mindy finds, people often respond badly to people who are realistic. "They think they're not being positive enough," she adds.

Approaches Are Very Individual

Attitudes toward life-threatening situations are not one-size-fits all, says Mindy. What works for one person may only make things more difficult for someone else.

Mindy learned this lesson the hard way. The first time she had breast cancer, she thought about the earliest example she'd ever had of somebody coping with crisis. That was her father struggling with an illness. "Everybody thought he was going to die, but he didn't," Mindy says.

She tried to learn coping techniques from her father. "My father used to tell us in detail of how he would look at me and he would look at my brother and he would think of all the things he needed to live for," she says. "He wanted to see us get married; he wanted to watch my brother's bar mitzvah."

The technique worked for her father, so Mindy tried to emulate it when she was faced her own life-threatening situation. When she started to worry about the breast cancer, she would stare at her sons, Max and Isaac, and think about her hopes for their futures. "Immediately I would throw myself into a pillow in my bedroom and start to bawl. Because, for me, thinking of all the things I wanted to live for meant thinking about all the things I was afraid of losing."

In other words, the approach backfired. "Instead of giving me strength, it was making me cry. And after like the ten millionth time I bolted from the room, I finally realized that maybe this approach wasn't working so well for me; maybe I needed to find a different approach." Effective methods of handling crises don't run in the family. Just because something worked for her dad didn't mean it would be equally effective for Mindy. She needed to find her own approach to life after cancer.

It's not always so easy, though, to figure out what works for you. As with other psychological issues, it's probably easier to analyze the past than the present, suggests Mindy. So, think about what coping techniques have worked for you in the past. Think about how you have responded to crises in the past—and what made you feel better, proposes the onco-psychologist.

Sometimes it helps, as it did with Mindy and her dad's approach, to also think about what doesn't work. Mindy learned that thinking about events she wanted to be present for would only upset her. In other words, she learned what *not* to do.

"Sometimes you just know from having a bad reaction, you can think—what was it that gave me that bad reaction Tuesday? What was going on that made me feel so bad?" says Mindy "Or, think 'I had such a fabulous day yesterday—what do I think was making me feel so good?'"

In the end, there are benefits to both positive thinking and realistic approaches. Optimism helps you dream big. Realism helps you get there. The goal is to pay attention to your own reactions and use the approaches that feel most natural and work best for you.

The same is true when it comes to superstition. Some people hear about my hospital gowns and think I'm nuts. Other people heard that I was writing a book about life after cancer, a project that didn't faze me, and worry that I was just asking for trouble. (Of course, they turned out to be right, but don't let them know; there's nothing as annoying as someone who says, "I told you so.") The bottom line is that these sorts of superstitions only "work" if you think they will, on some level. So don't beat yourself up: chances are, your superstitions are providing emotional support. The key is to find the coping style that works for you and stick with it.

What to Do about It

There are other ways to deal with anxiety and depression beyond analyzing and applying your own psychological processes. You don't have to just accept it. The Wellness Issues section of the book offers a wide range of approaches, and you can pick the one or ones that work best for you. Every cancer survivor should think hard about exercise and nutrition. These are the two areas where you can make a real difference in your chances of recurrence or another cancer and, just as important, improve your quality of life.

In addition, there is East Asian medicine, an entire system discussed in chapter 13, which incorporates

- Acupuncture
- Herbal therapy
- Physical manipulation
- Qigong

There are also a host of alternate modalities. Chapter 15 discusses the following:

- Natural products (such as vitamin supplements and probiotics)
- Mind and body medicine (including meditation, guided imagery, and journaling)
- Manipulative and body-based practices (think about massage therapy and yoga)
- Psychosocial support (which includes support groups and individual therapy)

These lists are far from exhaustive. Talk to your friends and family, health-care providers, and therapists. Ask them what techniques have been helpful for them. There's much to explore, and different approaches may help at different parts of your post-cancer journey.

Frequently Asked Questions

Q: I'm feeling more sad and anxious now than I was when I was first told I had cancer, or during the whole treatment process. Is that normal?

A: Absolutely. When you're going through treatment, you're very busy, and you're actively fighting the disease. Once you're done, you have more time on your hands. For most people, this is when you really start to have an emotional response.

Q: I'm nervous, but feeling positive. I have a feeling I am done with cancer. But a friend of mine tells me I'm fooling myself. Am I?

A: If you've followed all the medical protocols that were advised and you are focusing on nutrition, exercise, and other activities to stay healthy, you're doing the right thing(s). Being a glass-half-full person is often helpful and can provide physical and psychological benefits. The big problem is when people you care about blame you for not being more realistic; just listen to your heart.

Q: But what about me? I think I'm being realistic, but my friends tell me I'm too pessimistic. Am I really hurting myself?

A: A realistic attitude is also very healthy. The key, again, is to follow all the appropriate medical protocols and focus on healthy living. Optimism isn't necessarily better for you than realism. The big problem is when people you care about blame you for not being more optimistic; just listen to your heart.

Q: I find I'm more superstitious than I used to be. Am I hurting myself? Am I on my way to becoming obsessive-compulsive?

A: As long as you're following the medical protocol and are prepared to deal with the consequences of your superstitions—whether it means doing laundry more often or paying for a certain item— you're probably not doing any harm. In fact, there are often benefits to following your superstition, though those tend to be more psychological than "magical." And, based on what we know today, there's no reason to think that having a superstition or two will lead you to OCD behavior.

Chapter 4

Sexuality and Intimacy

Elissa Bantug was first diagnosed with breast cancer when she was twenty-three years old. Two years later, she had a recurrence, followed by a bilateral mastectomy. So by the tender age of twenty-five, when Elissa was barely out of graduate school, she'd lost months of her life, two breasts, and her strawberry blond hair.

"Right after treatment, I was in a new relationship and my sex life was terrible," says Elissa. "There were days when I was feeling so broken and so unfeminine and so unhappy with my body."

She just wanted to feel whole, and part of that had to do with sexuality. She wanted to be held; she wanted to be told she was beautiful and desirable. "I tried to engage my boyfriend in going to bed," she remembers. "He looked at me like I was crazy. He said he wanted to give me space to heal." Space was the last thing Elissa wanted.

Of course, Elissa's boyfriend was thinking that she was fragile. He was scared that he might hurt her. He worried that being intimate would interfere with her treatments or possibly sap the last little bit of energy she had. He was trying to give her exactly what he thought she needed.

Unfortunately, it wasn't what she wanted.

"I was really angry, and we had this awful, awful fight, probably seventy-two hours post-mastectomy," Elissa remembers. "I was like, 'You don't love me,'" Elissa remembers telling her boyfriend. "I just needed him to tell me that I was beautiful and that he'd love me no matter what."

When they did, finally, have sex, it was awkward. Elissa's boyfriend was very nervous and didn't know what to do. He didn't know where to touch—what might hurt and what might draw attention to scars and make Elissa feel self-conscious.

For Elissa's part, she wanted to be intimate, but her body wasn't cooperating. "I was like, 'Why isn't my body doing what I need it to do? Why do I have no sex drive? Why can I not have my body perform the way I want it to?'" she asks. "It was really, really frustrating."

Elissa felt betrayed by her own body. "I had had a very healthy sex life before I had cancer," she says. "I felt like cancer had robbed me of so much. This was one area that I needed to have twenty or thirty minutes to feel whole again and not to think about cancer," she says. Unfortunately, it didn't work out that way.

Alas, she's not alone.

Sexual problems are one of the most common—and disturbing— effects of cancer and treatment.[1] The National Cancer Institute reports that more than 40 percent of cancer survivors experience some sort of sexual dysfunction. Anne Katz, RN, PhD, adjunct professor at the University of Manitoba in Winnipeg and sexuality counselor at CancerCare Manitoba, puts that figure at about 80 percent of all cancer survivors. Sexual difficulties hit survivors of

---

1. Anne Katz, *Breaking the Silence on Cancer and Sexuality: A Handbook for Healthcare Providers* (Pittsburgh: Oncology Nursing Society, 2007), 15.

breast cancer, prostate cancer, and people with hematological cancers after bone marrow stem cell transplants especially hard, says Katz.

It's almost always the treatment, not the cancer itself, that causes the problems. The only exceptions are some brain cancers. If, for instance, someone has a pituitary tumor, the tumor itself will have an effect on sex hormone production. But otherwise, the culprit is surgery, chemotherapy, radiation, or hormone treatment. In other words, most people are just fine, until they actually try to get better.

Sexual problems tend to have an enormous effect on our quality of life. They can seem insurmountable, too, and they aren't very easy to treat. One reason is that a lot of people don't feel comfortable discussing sexual dysfunction with their onco docs. Talking about sex is awkward enough to discuss at the best of times, much less with someone you barely know, someone you have a very clinical relationship with. "There's this hesitancy to bring up sexual problems," Katz says, "because, frankly, health-care providers come with the same cultural and religious baggage their patients do." Sex ed was awkward in high school, and it hasn't gotten any less so with the years.

Besides, when a doctor just devoted months or more to saving your life, it seems a little, oh, embarrassing to say, I want to live *and* I want to orgasm.

"It's really a multi-factorial problem," says Leslie Shrover, PhD, professor in the Department of Cancer Prevention and Population Sciences at the University of Texas MD Anderson Cancer Center. Typically, intimacy problems are mind-body issues and demand attention on psychological, relational, and cultural levels. They may require medical treatment, information, and emotional support. Often, having another set of eardrums focused on your concerns can help you sort them out.

The first step is to talk with a professional and try to dissect the various issues involved. Once you can figure out the component parts of the problem—be they difficulties with arousal, performance, or orgasm—you can tackle each component, one at a time.

Some hospitals have programs devoted to the topic. At Memorial Sloan-Kettering, for instance, there's a Female Sexual Medicine and Health Program that enables survivors to sit with a psychologist, a gynecologist, and a nurse practitioner. (Alas, it's for women only.) But even as gender-discriminatory as the program is, it's still more support than is typically available to the average cancer patient or survivor.

Low Libido

Surgery seems to have been Elissa's problem, but it's not the only type of cancer treatment that can cause people to lose their sex drive. Anyone on hormone therapy—including men who've been treated for prostate cancer or women who've had breast or ovarian cancer—as well as anyone who's been through a bone marrow transplant or stem cell therapy is at risk.

Treatment isn't the only potential culprit in sexual dysfunction, either. There are all sorts of emotional issues involved. The diagnosis of cancer itself, for starters, is enough to make you distrust your body. It let you down in the doctor's office or CT scan room, after all, so who's to say it can hold its own in bed?

Surgery, chemotherapy, radiation, and hormone therapy aren't exactly easy on flesh and bone, either. Survivors experience all sorts of psychological after-effects ranging from poor body image, pain, and fatigue to depression, anxiety, and stress.

All those pills don't help, either: antidepressants, anti-anxiety meds, pain medication, anti-nausea pills, and so on. You name a type of medication and, chances are, some cancer survivor is popping it daily. Lots of us have enough medication to set up our own pharmacies. None of this encourages a good roll in the hay.

Sometimes survivors, like Elissa, notice that they're "not so into it" anymore. Sometimes it's the partner who—hopefully with great tact and sensitivity—has pointed out the change. Or perhaps a single person might observe that he or she isn't dating anymore; what would be the point of risking rejection, when being intimate doesn't sound all that appealing anyway?

No matter how the issue comes to light, though, it's more than a little awkward and uncomfortable. As Elissa points out, it's just one more thing that cancer takes from us. Freud has been discredited, but I'm with him on one thing: work and sex are key to enjoying life.

Every so often, there's a magic pill that does the trick. Viagra, for instance, is often very effective with erectile dysfunction. Most of the time, though, low libido is a multi-faceted and very frustrating predicament. When you're experiencing an emotional cocktail of depression, stress, anxiety (garden-variety and performance-specific), fear (of recurrence, rejection, or something else), hot flashes, fatigue, nausea, and pain, not to mention worries about your partner or your body image, it's amazing anyone *ever* has sex after cancer treatment.

Follow Your Partner

Katz suggests that we should rethink how desire fits into our vision of the human sexual response cycle. "A lot of people assume that desire or libido is the first thing" to focus on, she says. "They assume that you have to feel desire before doing anything." But that's not necessarily true, she adds. "There's been a lot of work that suggests that, particularly for women, that's actually not the case," Katz adds.

Instead of just sitting around waiting for your libido to kick in, suggests Katz, maybe women should follow their partners' sexual appetite. Then, assuming that the atmosphere—time, place, and mood—is appropriate, and the sexual stimulation is exciting, Katz suggests, desire may result.[2] Go with the flow, in other words, and it might take you where you want to be. Lesbian couples may well have a distinct advantage over others. Katz isn't convinced this approach works as well with men.

---

2. Katz, *Breaking the Silence*, 15.

Onco-sexuality counselors like Katz can sometimes help couples sort out these issues and improve their sex lives. "I'm quite clear I can't solve a patient's problem," Katz says of her part in the process. "I'm not the Sex Police, who will come around to your house at 10:20 on a Saturday evening to see how you're doing. All I can do is give someone the tools and the information: 'Here's what has helped other people, why not try it?'"

Arousal and desire are two completely different issues, explains Katz. "Desire is a brain-heart thing," she says. "Arousal is a physical thing that also has associated cerebral manifestations. Arousal for men is about erection; arousal for women is about lubrication." Arousal isn't necessarily related to desire or sex drive, though; the two can operate differently, she explains. The body can react, occasionally, regardless of what the mind is up to. "Sometimes it's about trying, about being in physical contact with someone," says Katz. "Sometimes there is reactive desire as opposed to spontaneous desire," she says.

Body Image

Yael was about to see her boyfriend for the first time after her lumpectomy, and she was nervous. Sure, she looked fine dressed. Her breast surgeon had done a beautiful job. No weird bumps, nothing lopsided. Her left breast was a little smaller than it had been, a tad more petite than the right. Did that matter? Yael wasn't sure.

She was pretty sure, though, that the surgery would become glaringly obvious as soon as she took off her bra. Sam used to like her breasts. He would suck on them and fondle them. There was no way he wouldn't notice a thick red line. Why hadn't she fallen for a nearsighted guy?

As it turned out, though, Sam was great. Gently and encouragingly, he said, "Let me kiss it and make it better." Then he proceeded to do just that. When Yael looked at her scar in the mirror the next day, she could swear it had gotten just a little bit smaller, just a little bit less intensely red.

Had Yael been fretting unnecessarily? The jury is still out. Some experts, such as MD Anderson's Shrover, think that she was.

"Not everyone worries about body image," says Shrover. "They've done studies and if you have a young, very attractive woman who gets breast cancer and they've always really prided themselves on how pretty they look, a small change like a scar on the breast may be more devastating to them than to an older woman having a mastectomy and deciding not to do reconstruction," she says. "Body image is very much dependent on what you expect and what you think your partner expects." Perhaps Yael just got a compliment?

Part of Shrover's point is that body image isn't just about hair loss, a little bit of scarring, and some weight gain. Some people have it much worse than Yael. "The big issues are people who have part of their face missing," says Shrover. "Or people who have had neck cancer and end up with a laryngectomy." A total laryngectomy can leave a patient unable to speak without a prosthetic voice box and breathing through a stoma in the opening of the neck.

Many experts, though, see body image as a real concern for all sorts of survivors, including those who've had breast cancer. "I can't tell you how many people undergo surgery and say, 'I can't look at myself in the mirror right now,'" says Shari Goldfarb, MD, who works as a medical oncologist at Memorial Sloan-Kettering Cancer Center. "Or they say, 'I haven't let my husband see me without my shirt on since my surgery.'"

Fortunately for these survivors, Goldfarb points out, there's an odd sort of silver lining in the extended and multi-faceted treatment that cancer patients often undergo. "Right after surgery, there's a big impact on body image," says Goldfarb. People are often overwhelmed by all the changes to their bodies. Many patients, though, go through chemotherapy, radiation, and sometimes additional surgery. "It gives them a good six to nine months while they are going through other treatments, before they start thinking about how other people will react," Goldfarb adds. During this time, survivors are healing both their physical and emotional scars. We also get a basis for comparison. As bad as it looks now, it used to be worse, and that can be comforting.

It seems to me that what this controversy suggests is that when you get right down to it, whether you're worried about your body image or not, your reaction is perfectly normal. It's nice to know, I think, that you're neither crazy nor all alone when it comes to such a personal issue.

Your New Body

The first step, before worrying about other people's reactions, is for survivors to come to terms with the "new you." "For each person," suggests Goldfarb, "it takes a different amount of time to come to terms with the new body. Time and counseling are often very helpful."

Katz advises many of these people. "It's really difficult; there's certainly not a one-size-fits-all solution," she says. "Sometimes it's a matter of reframing and helping people understand that we judge our own bodies much more harshly than anybody else does," she adds.

People starting a new relationship have a bit of an advantage. "Lust really does put blinders on people," says Katz. "When, in that part of the relationship at the beginning where it's really lustful, people will see past the changes, or, when you're really into someone, you don't have to think about that kind of stuff. You want to get with someone."

Of course, that's not true for all couples. "It has more to do with younger relationships than younger people," says Katz. In other words, a fifty-year-old who is dating has more in common with a twenty-year-old who's dating than a long-married, thirty-something survivor. "Sometimes it's worse [for older people] because there's sometimes baggage, more baggage, as we get older," Katz notes. Wrinkles and gray hair do take a toll. "People might not be that confident in their bodies," she adds.

It's not always easy to feel comfortable with your post-treatment body. Look at it, admire it, touch it, the experts say. I have to admit, it took me a few days before I could touch my mastectomy scars. They looked so tender and vulnerable. I had an irrational fear that somehow I could rip them open. It took even longer before I could clean off the marks left by the bandage adhesives.

Once I worked up the nerve to touch the scars, though, I was able to convince myself that the breasts—really the nipple-less boob mounds made from my thighs because, inexplicably, there wasn't enough fat in my stomach—were mine. When I had to clean and bandage the drain scars, it was simultaneously a little icky and a little surprising. I'd had both my boobs chopped off, but somehow I couldn't see what I was doing because there were these *things* in the way.

For some breast cancer survivors, reconstruction is central to adjusting to their new bodies. "I woke up with breast mounds so I didn't look down and see a concave chest," says Beth (not me), who also had a double mastectomy and reconstruction when she was in her forties. "I think that that made a world of difference." She remembers feeling totally calm, completely comfortable with her post-surgery body from the moment she laid eyes on it. "If I had woken up to a concave chest with scars, it would have been different," she is certain.

Others need to put a little more effort into reclaiming their bodies.

To do this, some experts recommend focusing on other parts of your body that weren't affected by treatment. After I finished treatment for Hodgkin's disease, which left me with three surgical scars around my neck, I started wearing turtlenecks that simultaneously hid the scars and showed off my breasts. Fortunately, the neck scars have faded now, so it's back to focusing on cleavage. These days, I don't wear anything that's tight enough to suggest that my breasts aren't quite "done" yet.

Others recommend having a pleasant experience, just you and your new bod. Try a warm bath, perhaps with some nice-smelling bubble bath. Or explore your new body by candlelight. Whatever you do, avoid the combination of fluorescent lighting and mirrors; in my opinion, the yellowish light adds a good ten years to anyone's appearance. Then touch yourself gently to get to know all your bumps and wrinkles. You can even start out exploring your body with your eyes closed. Just make sure you don't knock that candle over; you've already spent enough time in the hospital. Just because you know all the nurses and orderlies is no reason to head back there.

It can help to explore your body solo before sharing it with someone else. You may find that different things excite or annoy you. And a little "don't squeeze that" warning is probably preferable to an ear-splitting shriek. That's equally true for men and women.

After my bilateral breast reconstruction, for instance, my plastic surgeon told me to be careful about taking hot showers or spilling cups of coffee on my chest; you lose feeling there and apparently can't always tell when something is too hot. "Some people end up with third-degree burns," he told me. The unanticipated benefit is that I don't mind taking the last shower in the morning, as I've been sticking with lukewarm water anyway. By touching myself, though, I learned—most important—what doesn't hurt.

Masturbation and even using a vibrator can help you figure out what brings you pleasure and can revive your interest in sex. Once you're more familiar with your "new body," you can direct someone else on the best way to bring you pleasure. With a little bit of knowledge, communication, and luck, you can hopefully avoid the sort of awkward disappointment that Elissa and her boyfriend experienced. (Incidentally, with a little ingenuity and mutual patience, they worked it all out.)

When You're Ready to Share

It may sound counter-intuitive, but Goldfarb says that partners are usually less upset about the body changes than the survivor is. Yael's boyfriend, for instance, took one look and told her, "You're still a beautiful woman."

"Sometimes you run into a partner who cannot deal with your body," Goldfarb adds. "But that says more about the partner than about you." Do you really want to be with someone who is so insecure and superficial that they can't appreciate your strength and beauty? The truth of the matter, in Goldfarb's experience, is that the most painful body image issues have to do with the survivor's own fear of acceptance, rather than with what the partners actually say or do.

If a couple has trouble re-connecting, sometimes it helps to spend a few hours enjoying each other's company without sex. Try a date night at the movies, or maybe an afternoon picnic with champagne and strawberries. Experts say this might help recapture your intimacy, your connection as a couple.

It's easiest, though, when couples feel as though they can talk about their fears and concerns. When Elissa couldn't have an open discussion with her boyfriend, for instance, they both ended up feeling frustrated. On the other hand, if you can share your intimacy, and your thoughts and feelings, it's an important step to rebuilding your relationship after cancer. Again, it might help for a couple to avail itself of a good therapist.

Performance Problems

"I was impotent for, I think, about eighteen months after my treatment," says Matthew Zachary, brain cancer survivor and founder of Stupid Cancer, the world's largest support organization for young adult cancer survivors. "I was completely emasculated."

Matthew, who was diagnosed at the age of twenty-one, found his life turned upside down by his diagnosis. He was told he might not regain some of his fine motor skills. He was told there was no treatment that could help. He was offered no physical therapy for his hand, no sexual counseling for his impotence. "That would have been nice," he says.

"I was single, and I refused to date because I didn't want to be in that situation," says Matthew. "Why would you enter a relationship if you're impotent and you're twenty-two?" Rather than set himself up for rejection, he just avoided the issue altogether.

When Matthew finally got up the nerve to try to date, it didn't go well. "The one time that I had disclosed what I had gone through to a friend, someone I was interested in, she broke down hysterically crying," Matthew remembers. Not exactly the most romantic gesture ever. "So I just stayed away from it for a while."

With considerable time, patience, and determination, Matthew was able to rehabilitate his hand on his own. He started out playing piano with just his right hand, then occasionally hitting a single note with his left. He worked patiently and consistently. "Music was such a powerful tool for me to express myself and just get it out, get it out of my system and figure out a way to make sense of the madness in a weird way," he says. Matthew's determination stood him well. It took a while, but eventually he started giving concerts and put out a few CDs.

Matthew was lucky when it came to his sexuality as well. After a while, he was no longer impotent, but he still had the physical scars of survivorship. After his first experience sharing his story, he chose to be upfront from the start. "I just decided to wear it on my sleeve, and if someone didn't like it, they could . . ." Matthew says. "It's as straightforward as 'I'm an open book, and, like it or not, this is who I am and you have no choice. Love me or hate me,'" Matthew explains. Did it work? Well, he's now married and has twin preschoolers. "It's been amazing, transformative, and has given me new purpose," he says.

Performance problems are more common than you think. Research shows that after treatment, between 20 percent and 30 percent of breast cancer survivors and nearly 80 percent of prostate cancer survivors, for instance, experience some sexual difficulties.[3]

---

3. Carol DeSantis et al., "Cancer Treatment and Survivorship Statistics," *CA: A Cancer Journal for Clinicians* 62 (2012): 213–277.

Men who have difficulty getting an erection have a number of options, according to MD Anderson Cancer Center.[4] The first line of attack for erectile dysfunction (ED) is usually PDE5 inhibitors, which often work. In addition to medications, there are vacuum erection devices, also known as vacuum construction devices, that fit over the penis and use suction to create an erection. Specially made latex bands or rings can help a man maintain his erection, though they should be used with care and never for more than thirty minutes at a time. Health-care providers can determine the best approach for each individual person.

Many men, and their partners, expect the same performance as in their twenties. Unfortunately, comorbidities and other issues unrelated to cancer may make that unlikely. While many women report that ED isn't a problem for them as long as there's hugging, kissing, and other signs of affection, men often feel unsatisfied without penetration, according to Anne Katz, RN, PhD, adjunct professor at the University of Manitoba in Winnipeg and sexuality counselor at CancerCare Manitoba, Canada. Women, on the other hand, are more distressed by lack of communication. If couples can communicate honestly and openly about their feelings, though, they have a better chance.

"I think that, unfortunately, we have all these different treatments that urologists prescribe," says Shriver, "from pills to injections into the penis to vacuum pumps to surgery to put in a penile prosthetic," she says. But often, notes Shriver, these don't do the trick.

"Part of it is because the partner's never involved" in the process. "You need to counsel the couple in how to use these things optimally," she adds. "Treatment with even brief counseling is so much better than just handing a guy a prescription."

---

4. "Sexuality and Your Cancer Treatment," *MD Anderson Cancer Center*. last modified February 21, 2012, http://www2.mdanderson.org/app/pe/index. cfm?pageName=opendoc&docid=852.

When Sex Is Painful

Women have a wider range of physical problems associated with sexual performance. Often the biggie is pain. There's nothing less sensual than feeling like someone rammed a jackhammer into your insides. Once a woman has felt that kind of pain, she's apt to be more tentative the next time around.

Sometimes the pain comes from vaginal dryness, which can be caused by chemotherapy, hormone treatment, and especially aromatase inhibitors, says Shrover. Fortunately, there are lots of lubricants available in pharmacies as well as in specialty shops. Go for either water- or silicone-based, but avoid perfumed or warming lubes, as they can cause allergic reactions. Oil-based lotions, such as petroleum jelly or baby oil, can increase chances of vaginal infection, notes MD Anderson Cancer Center.[5] Also, shy away from anything with parabens (often listed as methylparaben, butylparaben, propylparaben, or benzylparaben, according to the Livestrong Foundation), which have been linked to increased cancer risk for both males and females.[6]

Here, too, working together as a couple is most effective, says Shrover. Some people are uncomfortable using lubricants with their partners; it feels like, if not an out-and-out failure, at least an embarrassment. So they may apply the lube in the bathroom before sex. But lubricants work best when applied repeatedly, as needed. (The subtle advanced preparation approach probably won't work for long.) Lubricants aren't solo affairs; the most effective way to deal with vaginal dryness is to incorporate the lube into your lovemaking.

---

5. "Vaginal Dryness," *MD Anderson Cancer Center*. last modified February 27, 2012, http://www2.mdanderson.org/app/pe/index.cfm?pageName=opendoc&doc id=1973.

6. Tacon, A.M. "What Are the Side Effects of Parabens?" *Livestrong Foundation*. last modified October 27, 2013, http://www.livestrong.com/article/194949-what-are-the-side-effects-of-parabens/.

If a woman has had a few painful experiences with intercourse—or even if she's just feeling nervous about it—she may involuntarily tense her muscles around the vaginal entrance, says Shriver. That, of course, causes more pain. So sometimes it is a matter of learning to control and relax those muscles.

Another option is vaginal moisturizers. We use facial moisturizers and body moisturizers all the time to make sure our skin is well hydrated. But somehow we never think about internal issues. Yet, according to Pure Romance, a purveyor of relationship and intimacy aids, about 40 percent of menopausal women experience vaginal dryness.[7]

Many women use the product, injecting vaginal moisturizers into their vagina with a tampon-like applicator every day for a week or week and a half until they see their symptoms decrease. Then they might use it two or three times a week for maintenance. Vaginal moisturizers can also prevent vaginal and yeast infections, according to Pure Romance.[8]

Pain that's not related to vaginal dryness could be vaginal atrophy, says Goldfarb. According to MD Anderson, that could result from certain types of pelvic surgery including a radical hysterectomy, or bladder or colon surgery. That could mean the vagina has become narrower or it has lost its elasticity.

Often, women with vaginal atrophy can benefit from physical therapy, pelvic floor therapy, and dilator therapy, says Goldfarb. Dilators for this purpose typically come in multiple sizes; you start small and work your way up from there, step by step. This process doesn't just facilitate intercourse; sometimes women need to use vaginal dilators just to enable gynecologists to conduct routine vaginal and cervical exams. Again, please consult with a health-care professional for instructions specific to your situation.

---

7. "What is Vaginal Moisturizer," *Pure Romance*. last modified November 4, 2009, http://pattybrisben.com/?s=vaginal+dryness+and+40%25.

8. Ibid.

Exercising the Pelvic Floor

Another topic, which people are reluctant to talk about, is incontinence, which is becoming more and more of an issue these days. "A lot of operations can cause chronic diarrhea or urinary leakage that's very difficult to control and happens during sex as well," says Shriver. An ostomy, for instance, refers to the surgically created opening in the body for the discharge of body wastes.

"There's no faster way to end somebody's sex life than if they're embarrassed by that." There's not much that can be done medically for this condition, so the key is working with your partner, she explains.

In addition, some experts suggest being careful about the amount of food and drink before a date. Change your ostomy pouch, even if it is less than one-third full; and make sure the ostomy bag is empty, flat, and out of the way. And, of course, try different positions until you find one that works.

Kegel Exercises

Kegel exercises can help both women and men improve bladder control. In fact, many doctors recommend them to women after childbirth for just that reason. They can be useful throughout your life.

Start by locating the pelvic floor muscles, which you can do by cutting off the flow of urine when you're peeing. The muscles you used for that are the ones you want to strengthen, the ones you will contract doing Kegel exercises. The exercise isn't complicated; there are just a few steps:

1. Contract the pelvic floor muscles (which you found earlier).
2. Hold this contraction for three seconds, then rest for three seconds.
3. Repeat ten times.

4. Work your way up to holding the contraction for ten seconds each time.

The goal is to be able to hold the contraction for ten seconds, then relax for ten seconds. Repeat the whole process ten times, preferably three times a day for maximum benefit.

While Kegels are essentially intended to aid with incontinence, there's a bonus: they can increase women's orgasms and improve men's erections.

Difficulty with Climaxing

Reaching orgasm can be more of a problem as we get older. But, surprisingly, cancer survivors don't usually have any more problems than anyone else, says Shrover. "It is relatively rare for cancer treatment to really damage the nerves that are involved in being able to feel the sensation of orgasm." More often difficulties stem more from stress and anxiety than from anything physical.

Men do sometimes experience dry orgasms, the psychologist says. That's when a man reaches climax, but does not ejaculate. "Sometimes men aren't warned about that and they're really upset and don't understand what happened," says Shrover. Also, she adds, men don't always know that they can have an orgasm without a firm erection, so they don't even try. Their partners can feel rejected, and that can lead to an unhappy cycle.

Women typically have fewer problems with orgasm after cancer treatment, says Shrover. "It's less common that there are changes in how and what kinds of stimulation help them reach orgasm." The major culprit is more likely to be pain, she says.

Matthew had the right idea, according to MD Anderson. It's best to resume sex when you're feeling ready; don't rush yourself. Sometimes the best way to start is to take it slow. Cuddle on the sofa, kiss, touch gently. Then, when you're ready, you can keep going.

Dating

"I've gone on so many dates it's ridiculous," says twenty-six-year old Khit, a two-time cancer survivor. "It's very rare that I get a second date after people find out that I had cancer," she says. And they find out pretty early on. Khit volunteers regularly for Imerman Angels and wears Imerman Angel gear every day. "People always ask, 'What is Imerman Angels?' or 'Are you a survivor?' So when I'm on a date with somebody, they know I'm a cancer survivor."

"My friends advise me that I shouldn't tell them so much at the beginning," says Khit. "But that's who I am. People should know right away that that's what I'm about." Another problem is that people tend to assume, when they hear she had vulval cancer, that Khit can't have children. "Some people don't even bother to ask me that because we're on date one, and talking about kids isn't really something you talk about on date one." So, they just make assumptions. And the response? "They still text me and say 'hi,' but they don't want to go on another date," says Khit.

Rachel's got her own horror story. After she was diagnosed with stage-three breast cancer at age twenty-four, she started dating a guy from the company where she works. "Everyone at my job knew that I had cancer because they had done a couple of fundraisers for me." So she didn't have to break the news to the guy, which made it easier.

"He said, 'I like you regardless; I want to give this a shot and help you through things.'" Rachel was thrilled and thought he would be a dependable source of support. "I thought he was a really good guy because he was willing to hop into a situation like that," she remembers. "It was amazing because most guys around that age, twenty-three or twenty-four, are like, 'Yeah, right, like I'm going to sit in on Friday nights with a girl who has cancer treatments and can't do anything,'" she adds.

The relationship started out really well. "It was kind of a distraction—you know that feeling when you're happy all the time" at a start of a relationship? Rachel was glad that she had something to focus on other than the cancer diagnosis and chemotherapy treatment. "It really helped me for the first month or two," Rachel remembers. "And then, as I started to lose my hair and my physical appearance changed, I felt his attitude change toward me as well," she says. Her energy level dropped, and she was no longer up for going to bars until two o'clock in the morning.

After Rachel finished chemo and found out she would need radiation treatment as well, the guy bailed. "He ended up saying that he couldn't give me everything that he thought I needed through this process," Rachel explains.

"It was horrible," says Rachel. "It was heartache in the middle of all this other crap. It was just an unnecessary addition of sadness to a process that was horrible already." Rachel had to deal with the loss of her hair, her energy, one of her breasts, and a boyfriend that she'd had good reason to believe would really be there for her.

When it comes to starting a new relationship during or after treatment, it helps to remember that dating is often anxiety-provoking, regardless of health status. You don't know if you'll feel a connection—or if the other person will. Even without appearance-altering cancer treatments, you may wonder if you look good, and if there have been changes to your body, you may have even less faith in your appearance. You may not know what you'll talk about, who will pay, and how the date will end. You may not even know how you *want* it to end. Then, of course, there's the whole issue of mind-reading, which has never been my forte.

Add to this awkward situation the element of cancer survivorship and it becomes even more fraught. Most survivors think, who's going to want me? Will I be physically up to it? Am I prepared to deal with rejection when I'm already feeling fragile?

How do you do it?

It helps to feel more confident in your body, but of course you can't click your heels three times and feel at home in your treatment-altered physique. You may have to pay some attention to yourself first. Nice-smelling lotions, a new hairstyle, makeup, or a new shirt might help. Try good posture and calm, deep breathing. If you can exude confidence, you might start to believe it yourself.

Have a little faith in yourself. Don't assume that your date will automatically reject you when he or she finds out about the cancer. Remember, other people have their own health issues, and those only increase as we get older—diabetes, heart disease, sexually transmitted diseases such as HIV. Even something that's not life-threatening, such as adult acne, can put a crack in your confidence. Somehow, though, people don't worry about dating with diabetes; if blood glucose levels drop while you're sitting there having a cup of coffee, someone with diabetes could become disoriented or even faint—right there, at the table. Talk about an awkward ending to a date.

Chances are, you'll start out just chatting, looking for (and finding) common hobbies, comparable experiences, and similar character traits. Maybe you both grew up in the country or you both love hiking. I know I prefer people who can make me laugh. You don't have to discuss medical conditions right away; wait until you know whether the person is kind enough and interesting enough to deserve getting to know you better.

The key is to have the discussion after you've developed a level of trust—and before you end up in bed. Just as every person is individual, so is every dating situation. Trust your judgment. There are no "right answers," just an approach that works for you.

Some people plan out exactly how to break the news, while others play it by ear. If you're feeling nervous, you can pick a neutral place and a relaxed time to talk. You might even want to practice talking about it in front of a mirror. Most sex therapists recommend using technical terms instead of slang or euphemisms; a fifty-year-old who says "pee-pee" when he means penis, for instance, can be a real turn-off.

You might want to make sure to mention these issues when you broach the Big C issue:

- Your current health status and how you're feeling
- The possibility of recurrence; if it's pretty unlikely, make sure to mention that
- Any potential sexual problems, such as erectile dysfunction or vaginal dryness; you might also want to mention any activities that are pleasurable or those that cause discomfort, as it helps to temper bad news with good (X, Y, or Z hurts, but A, B, and C are really great)
- Any physical changes to your body, such as scars or burns, that might be visible in bed
- Your ability to have children

If your worst nightmare happens, if the person rejects you because of your medical history, then clearly that's not the kind of person you want in your life long-term. You deserve better. You've proven yourself to be strong, determined, and resilient. You want a partner who truly cares about you and who accepts you as you are.

That's what Rachel ultimately decided. "Now I can look back at it and say he was a jerk. He wasn't man enough for the situation, and he wasn't good enough for me because I turned out to be a really positive and put-together person, and he's missing out."

She doesn't look back on that relationship with regrets. "It was awful, but it helped me look for the right qualities in a guy after that—because I said to myself, I'm not going to fall for this again."

Rachel realized that she wanted a different kind of boyfriend, now that she's been through a life-threatening illness. "I knew that I needed a sense of maturity from a person I was going to date," she says. "I think before cancer, what I was looking for in guys was someone who was good looking, someone who liked to have a good time, someone who liked to go out, someone who had a bunch of friends." Mostly superficial qualities, she has since decided.

"After cancer, I started to look a little deeper; I started to look for maturity, making sure that he was capable of dealing with things that were serious, someone who was internally a good person," Rachel says. "When you're young, you're like, oh I just like to have fun, I just like to go out and drink." But that was no longer Rachel. Besides, these days, waking up with a hangover reminds her too much of chemotherapy. "It made me think that I need a partner, I need a support system. It's a totally different way of looking at things."

She's glad of the change in her attitude. "I think it's brought me a lot closer to a lot of friends, because we've made that deeper connection. Everything's different—and so much better. It's deeper and better and more fulfilling than just hanging out with people who go drinking and then have nothing to do with you afterward." It's a hard way to learn a lesson, but a good one. At least for Rachel.

The best part, for Rachel, is that she's found someone else. She was participating in the Susan G. Komen Three-Day for the Cure, a sixty-mile walk that raises money for breast cancer research and patient support programs. She was walking with seven friends on "Team Rach," and they ran into a guy who was doing the walk on his own, dressed in full fire gear.

"He started out walking with us and then stayed with us for the whole three days," says Rachel. He had no friends or family who'd had breast cancer; he just wanted to do something to fight the disease. He walked with twenty pounds of fire gear because he figured it was as close as he could come to experiencing what it must be like for cancer patients and survivors to do the walk.

This guy is mature, very giving, and really supportive of Rachel. And wherever she volunteers—the Komen Foundation, Living Beyond Breast Cancer, you name it—he gets involved, too. "I guess because he was overseas [in the Marines in Iraq] and he fights fire for a living, he kind of knows what it's like to have your life on the line," she says. In a way, he kind of understands what the cancer experience was like for Rachel. "It's a crazy love story," she says.

Focusing on Wellness

A number of the suggestions in the Wellness Issues section can help with sexual dysfunction as well. Exercise, for instance, can help you relax, strengthen your body, help you gain strength, and release endorphins. (For more about exercise, see Chapter 12: Exercise.) Proper nutrition (see Chapter 13: Nutrition) can improve your energy level and help you feel stronger and healthier. Therapy can help you sort out the issues and deal with them (see Chapter 15: Other Complementary Approaches; to track down organizations that can help, take a look at Appendix 1: Resources for Survivorship).

Sex helps us create and enhance connections with other people, gives pleasure, keeps us going as a human race, and helps us feel alive. It can be difficult to talk about, but it's worth it. A little talking, education, treatment, and bravery can go a long way. After all, one of the reasons you fought so hard to stay alive is to enjoy life again. And sexuality is an important part of that.

Frequently Asked Questions

Q: When can I have sex again after treatment?

A: Check with your doctor, but typically you can do it as soon as you're feeling up to it physically.

Q: I'm frustrated because my sex drive isn't what it used to be. (And I think my partner is frustrated, too.) What can I do?

A: Think about all the things you've been doing to your body— surgery, chemotherapy, and radiation, not to mention stress. The way you're feeling (or not feeling) is to be expected, all things considered. Give yourself some time to feel ready. If you're concerned, there may be several factors at work, so speak with a social worker or health-care professional to try to dissect the various components. Then work on them, one at a time. It's much less overwhelming that way.

Q: I'm worried about dating. My body is different than it was; will anyone want me?

A: Start taking steps toward feeling comfortable with your "new" body—small things such as hot baths, nice lotion, or a new shirt might help. Once you are more confident about your body, it will be much easier to share it with someone else. Remember: anyone who rejects you because of a scar probably isn't the kind of person you want to spend your life with, anyway.

Q: I've heard about Kegel exercises. What are they, and how do they help?

A: Kegel exercises aid with incontinence, improve women's orgasms, and improve men's erections. This chapter describes the process in more detail.

Q: What if my partner no longer wants me after I've been treated for cancer?

A: Anyone who doesn't appreciate your strength and beauty, as a cancer survivor and a person, isn't worth your time. There are better options out there.

Q: Does cancer treatment cause difficulties with orgasm?

A: Cancer treatment interferes with just about everything in your body. But orgasm isn't as much a problem as other types of sexual dysfunction. Sometimes men have dry orgasms. You can still make love, in other words, but you may have to modify some of your activities.

Chapter 5

Fertility

Tito, who was diagnosed with Hodgkin's Lymphoma at age seventeen, didn't think about fertility before he started cancer treatment. He was still in high school and wasn't thinking much beyond high school graduation. Being a child himself, the thought of having his own children didn't occur to Tito. Nor did it occur to his onco docs, who didn't even mention the possibility of banking his sperm.

Now that he's in his late twenties, Tito is in a serious relationship with a woman and is wondering what his future will hold. Will they get married—and will they be able to have children? "It's hard for a guy to talk about fertility with his girlfriend," he worries. It's difficult to tell someone you care about that you might not be able to start a family with her.

Joe had a different experience. He was diagnosed with a rare kind of non-Hodgkin's lymphoma when he was eighteen, a very fast-growing cancer. His doctors were concerned, and he was rushed immediately into chemotherapy treatment. "When I was admitted, they said that normally we would have you bank sperm, but we need you to start chemotherapy immediately," Joe remembers.

At the time, Joe didn't think about it. He was a kid himself, in his first semester at college; he wasn't worried about having his own child. But when he looks back on what happens, Joe is a little confused. "Really? There was no time? I was an eighteen-year-old kid," he says. All he needed was a little privacy and a cup.

The good news is that Joe is fine and now is married, with a healthy five-year-old daughter.

Ilana's cancer story involved fertility issues from the start.

Like Tito and Joe, Ilana's cancer was discovered when she was young and single. At age twenty-one, she was finishing her last year of college when she found out she had ovarian cancer. Because of a surprising (and lucky) bout of extreme pain near her appendix, she rushed to the local hospital emergency room, ended up being admitted, having a cyst removed from one of her ovaries, and being told to check with an oncologist for further testing.

She interviewed a few oncologists and ended up with a diagnosis of ovarian cancer, stage one. Ilana had surgery followed by several months of chemotherapy—yet she still managed to graduate from college on time.

Her doctor brought up the idea of fertility preservation, but her choices were pretty limited. At that point, 1994, technology had not yet developed to the place where you could freeze eggs unfertilized. And Ilana was single, with no sperm donor in sight. "I thought for a very brief week about which one of my guy friends I would ask to father my children," she remembers. "But I don't know that any twenty-one-year-old guy is prepared to answer that question on the fly—and do it on a week's notice." Fortunately, Ilana's oncologist thought her remaining ovary would be OK, so she decided not to do anything about her fertility just then.

Ilana's oncologist did warn her, "Once you find the right person, don't wait very long. Chemotherapy ages your ovary, and you only have one," he said. "So you'll need to get to it."

Ilana is nothing if not organized, and after a year of marriage, when she was thirty-six—giving herself a little time to get used to having a spouse before adding to the family mix—she and her husband began preparing to begin a family. She mentioned this to her oncologist, who recommended she get a baseline mammography because of her health history and because, once she got pregnant and started breastfeeding, she wouldn't have a mammo for a long time. "Why don't you go get a baseline mammogram," he said, "just to have it in the records, and then go and have babies."

That turned out to be a prescient suggestion, as the "routine" mammo turned up stage-two breast cancer. Fortunately, though, the cancer was unrelated to the ovarian; it was a second "new" cancer, not a recurrence. Always thorough in her research and decision making, Ilana got second and third opinions. They all said the same thing about her cancer and treatment, but only the second opinion, the oncologist at a local private hospital, mentioned fertility preservation. Ilana brought the idea back to her own oncologist, who was very supportive and helpful, even though she didn't mention the idea originally.

"That's the part that frustrates me," says Ilana. "I would love to help make it become the normal standard of care that oncologists say to all patients immediately, 'If you want to preserve your fertility, it has to be part of our treatment discussion starting now.'" Starting on the day of diagnosis.

"It's not the norm, and it really should be because the demographics are changing. More younger women are getting cancer and more older women are having children," says Ilana. "So the overlap now is greater than it used to be." In addition, more and more people are surviving cancer, which means that quality-of-life issues are becoming increasingly prominent for more and more people.

Enter Ilana's tightrope walk. She wanted to do everything she could to simultaneously preserve her fertility and her life. What would be the point of having a baby if she wouldn't be around to see it grow up? By the same token, Ilana had always known she wanted to be a mother, and she knew her life wouldn't be the same without that experience.

Ilana contacted the local fertility clinic, the one several of her friends had used. Normally it would have been a three-week wait for a consult, but because she told them she had cancer, she ended up with an appointment that very afternoon.

The oncologist and reproductive endocrinologist negotiated extensively about whether Ilana could delay cancer treatment for fertility preservation, and for how long. Ilana ended up doing one IVF cycle and retrieval immediately, then having a double mastectomy. While she rested up from surgery in preparation for chemotherapy treatment, Ilana did another round of IVF. It fit neatly into the schedule.

"Someone said to me, 'Are you sure you want to go through all the IVF stuff right after a double mastectomy?'" Ilana remembers. "I said, 'Are you kidding? After the mastectomy, this is nothing.'" Between the two IVF cycles, before and after the surgery, Ilana and her husband ended up with five frozen embryos.

But Ilana had to reconcile herself to not breastfeeding. It was difficult, but she thought, "at least I'll have a baby—and be alive to watch it grow up."

Next, Ilana came to realize that she wouldn't be able to carry the fetus. "It's not that I didn't want to—I would have loved to," she says. But she had a laundry list of complications: she was on Tamoxifen (which is known to cause birth defects), her tumor was estrogen receptor positive (which makes the elevated levels of hormones during pregnancy especially dangerous), and after everything her body had been through, in terms of cancer and its treatment, it wasn't clear whether her body could sustain a pregnancy.

Just because it was a logical decision, though, didn't make it an easy one. "It was hard because slowly, piece by piece, pregnancy was getting further and further away from me," says Ilana.

Shortly after she finished chemo, Ilana turned her attention to finding a gestational carrier for the pregnancy; this woman would carry the embryos created by Ilana's eggs and her husband's sperm, hopefully to term. Gestational carriers must be evaluated physically and emotionally for the role, according to the American Society for Reproductive Medicine. "We didn't have an obvious choice," she says. "I didn't have a sister, and my husband's sister didn't qualify because she didn't have children at that point."

"We decided this was not something we could ask someone to do," Ilana explains. "We have friends and relatives who we thought might be good candidates, but we could never ask someone to do this—no matter how many times we say, 'It's OK to say no,' it's too much pressure to put on a relationship." So they turned to a lawyer who specializes in fertility issues to find a carrier. But pretty soon, a friend of Ilana's and her husband spoke up and volunteered to do it. It was a huge process, emotionally, physically, and financially, and, ultimately, they used all five embryos.

None of them took; the friend never became pregnant despite already having children of her own. They never found out why. "We were all extremely disappointed. Happy we had gone through this together, but extremely disappointed," says Ilana.

Ilana and her husband began to explore other options, notably donor eggs and adoption, but the couple was turned down by several adoption agencies because of her medical history. "They said we weren't good candidates; they wouldn't work with us," Ilana explains. So Ilana and her husband started attending donor egg support groups and thinking seriously about donor eggs.

"The thing we saw was that when it comes to fertility issues, every couple hits a temporary road block at some point, and it's a different point for everyone," says Ilana. "My roadblock was when I thought the child wouldn't be biologically mine," she explains. "I'd always wanted children, and I'd worked so hard to preserve my fertility."

She really wanted to have a biological relationship with her children, if at all possible.

"I need to know I have no more eggs," she told her husband. So they went to speak with their fertility doctor, who had some reservations about the procedure.

"Look," he told the couple, "I'm not eager to put you through this physically. I'm not eager to put you through this financially. I have no faith that we will get any viable eggs out of you," he said. "But if you're telling me that this is the only way you're going to be emotionally able to move on, then I will agree to it."

Yes, that was what Ilana was saying.

So Ilana went off Tamoxifen temporarily and did a cycle of IVF. Then she had some necessary reconstructive surgery, which she couldn't do while on Tamoxifen. Again, it was a matter of accomplishing two medical procedures at the same time.

The doctor told her, "I don't know why your friend didn't work out, but we can't use her again." Ilana and her husband returned to the lawyer to start looking for a new carrier.

Ilana, ever the multi-tasker, ended up simultaneously recuperating from surgery, looking for another carrier, and going through one more round of IVF. Between the two cycles, one before and one after surgery, she and her husband ended up with two more frozen embryos.

The search began, then, all of a sudden, another friend, whom Ilana hadn't spoken with in years, volunteered to be a carrier. "She'd had two great pregnancies, she loved being pregnant, and she had always thought about being a carrier," says Ilana. "She said that when she heard we were looking, she knew it was *besheret*, it was meant to be, and her husband was immediately supportive," she adds.

They went through the whole process—the physical exams, the psych exams, and the legal arrangements. Then they inserted both embryos and crossed their collective fingers.

Ilana and company then had, finally, their storybook ending. Both embryos took. The carrier was carrying twins—a boy and a girl. The babies were born without incident a little early, but that's common for twins. They're healthy and beautiful and will never, ever wonder if they were truly wanted.

Effects of Cancer Treatment on Fertility

While cancer itself usually has no effect on fertility, treating the disease often does. The surgery, chemotherapy, radiation, and hormone treatments that can save our lives can make it hard for us to bring a new life into the world. When I talked with survivors about what topics they wanted to see in this book, fertility was often one of the first mentioned; having a family is an important part of life after cancer.

In many cases, once treatment is completed, most fertility decisions have been made de facto, which can add another burden for survivors. The best time, the most effective time, to think about fertility is before you start treatment.

Cancer treatments affect men's and women's fertility in different ways.

Women's Fertility

Every cancer has its own treatment protocol, and different types of treatments have varying effects on a woman's fertility. Specifically, surgical removal of the uterus or ovary causes permanent infertility. Total body irradiation comes pretty close, although according to MD Anderson Medical Center, a few young women have been able to have babies following that level of radiation treatment.[1] Other radiation treatments can damage a woman's ovaries and can increase

---

1. "Preserving Fertility Before Treatment," *MD Anderson Cancer Center*, accessed December 4, 2013, http://www.mdanderson.org/patient-and-cancer-information/cancer-information/cancer-topics/detection-and-diagnosis/preserving-fertility/index.html.

the risk of miscarriage, low-birth-weight infants, and premature births. In addition, bone marrow and cell transplants can stop a woman from releasing eggs, often permanently.

Other types of treatment have less clear-cut effects on reproduction. Chemotherapy damages eggs stored in the uterus, though the extent of the damage depends on the type and amount of chemo given. According to the American Cancer Society,[2] the types of chemo most likely to hurt fertility include

- Cyclophosphamide (Cytoxan)
- Ifosfamide (Ifex)
- Melphalan (Alkeran)
- Busulfan
- Procarbazine
- Chlorambucil (Leukeran)
- Carmustine (BCNU)
- Lomustine (CCNU)
- Mechlorethamine (Mustargen)

Many women emerge from cancer treatment in early menopause. In case you were wondering, menopause qualifies as "early" when it hits a woman before age forty. It can happen when both ovaries are removed, or sometimes with radiation or chemotherapy (notably alkylating agents, such as cyclophosphamide). In fact, it occurs so often with chemo that it's got its own nickname; many patients and survivors call chemotherapy-induced menopause "chemo-pause."

Women who get treatment before age thirty-five and those who receive lower doses of chemo or radiation are more likely to regain their periods as their bodies return to their "new normal," though there's no guarantee that menstruation will be regular again. I enjoyed both of those therapies and began menstruating again maybe six months after treatment.

2. "Treatments and Side Effects," *American Cancer Society*, accessed December 2, 2013, http://www.cancer.org/treatment/treatmentsandsideeffects/fertilityandcancerwhataremyoptions/fertility-and-cancer-information-women.

Even if your periods restart, though, it doesn't mean you'll be able to get pregnant, alas. Plus, you're at risk of early infertility and menopause because all or some of your eggs may have been damaged or killed outright during treatment. So much is uncertain about cancer treatment and fertility. But research is ongoing.

Effects on Men's Fertility

Men aren't immune from temporary or permanent infertility caused by cancer treatment. Surgical removal of the testicles causes infertility. High doses of radiation, especially to the testicles or brain, can eliminate all sperm cell-producing cells in the testicles or, at least, damage them. As with women, bone marrow and cell transplants can put an end to the ability to have kids.

In addition, certain types of surgery can affect a man's fertility. If both testicles have been removed, for instance, a man will not be able to produce sperm. But if only one testicle is removed, sperm production is possible, though it depends on the health of the remaining testicle. Some surgical treatments for prostate or bladder cancer can leave a man without sperm as well.

Some men with testicular cancer may well have been infertile before they were diagnosed. Sometimes cancer is underhanded that way. The good news, according to MD Anderson, is that about half of the men with testicular cancer who have one testicle removed can still recover some fertility.

Chemo is, of course, a culprit in male infertility as well as female. The higher the dose of chemotherapy, the longer it takes for the body to start producing maturing sperm cells. If sperm production hasn't recovered within four years, though, doctors worry that it is less likely to ever recover. But, don't give up hope; some men have regained their fertility as late as a decade from the end of treatment. Chemotherapy drugs that are linked to the highest risk of infertility in men, according to the American Cancer Society,[3] include

---

3. "Fertility and Cancer," *American Cancer Society*, accessed December 2, 2013, http://www.cancer.org/treatment/treatmentsandsideeffects/physicalsideeffects/ fertilityandcancerwhataremyoptions/fertility-and-cancer-cancer-treatment-fertility-men.

- Chlorambucil (Leukeran)
- Cyclophosphamide (Cytoxan)
- Procarbazine
- Melphalan (Alkeran)
- Cisplatin
- Nitrogen mustard
- Actinomycin D

Finally, some hormone therapies can affect a man's fertility. Really, so much of this varies from individual to individual that it's best to check with your doctor before starting treatment to find out whether—and how—it will affect your ability to have children.

Planning Ahead

Much of the time, the key to preserving fertility through cancer treatment involves planning ahead. Of course, as Ilana experienced, it is a delicate balance between saving your life and preserving your fertility. Fortunately, oncologists can guide you in making those decisions. It can help to talk with both an oncologist and a fertility specialist together.

Timing is really critical. Women's fertility is especially time-sensitive; as we age, it becomes harder and harder to get pregnant and carry it successfully. "If your doctor puts you on medication, on anti-estrogens, for three to five years or more," says Stephen R. Lincoln, MD, FACOG, medical director and co-founder of the Fertility Preservation Center for Cancer Patients at GIVF, "your ability to get pregnant can be naturally impaired."

Unfortunately, though, not enough cancer patients are told about the risks and possibilities before they begin treatment. Only about half of cancer patients talk with their oncologists about fertility, says Lincoln, but closer to 60 percent of women cancer patients want to have these discussions. In addition, a 2013 study by the American Society for Reproductive Medicine found that only 3 percent underwent fertility preservation.[4] That leaves a lot of cancer survivors who didn't preserve their options in advance, and are unclear about their fertility options.

One of the hidden advantages to thinking about fertility is that it can give a cancer patient or survivor a sense of control. "Cancer has taken away so much from patients," says Lauren Haring, BS, ASN, RN, who works extensively with cancer patients and survivors at the Genetics and IVF Institute. "This is something that they're making a conscious choice to do for themselves. It gives them a little bit of control over this unfortunate rollercoaster that they can't get off of."

The Nitty-Gritty Details

Cancer patients who take action before starting treatment have a couple of options for banking their vitals, just in case. Of course, not every option works for every patient; you should speak with an oncologist about what is appropriate for your situation.

Freezing Embryos. This is probably the most successful option for women, and fertility specialists have been doing it in the United States since the 1980s. The woman takes fertility drugs, often daily injections, to stimulate her ovaries to produce multiple eggs. These eggs are then fertilized with sperm from a partner or donor, and stored cryogenically.

Fertility specialists want to boost the number of eggs produced in hopes that they'll be able to retrieve more than one egg at a time. Simply put, human reproductive systems can be a little careless with those eggs. "We humans are not very efficient at reproduction," says Lincoln. "If you look at other animal species, like the deer or the rabbit, for example, they'll get pregnant with 90 percent of their

---

4.   ASRM Office of Public Affairs, "Fertility Preservation for Cancer Patients: Demographic Disparities in Counseling and Financial Concerns Are Barriers to Utilization," *The American Society for Reproductive Medicine*, October 23, 2012.

cycles, which is why the deer has one cycle a year. The rabbit may have three or four, but they'll have three or four litters a year." Compare that to us humans. Even during our prime reproductive age, in our twenties, our pregnancy rate is only about 20 percent to 25 percent a month. "That's why it requires multiple eggs to have a higher success rate," says Lincoln.

Fertility specialists are getting better at it. When they first started freezing and thawing eggs, it often took as many as one hundred eggs before achieving a successful delivery. But, says Lincoln, it only takes five to ten eggs now, on average, to make a baby. Ideally, fertility specialists try to get ten to fifteen mature eggs with each of these stimulation cycles, says Lincoln, though not everyone hits the mark.

Doctors remove the eggs just before ovulation using a needle inserted into the ovary through the vagina. They can be frozen as is or fertilized with sperm into embryos. Embryos can be stored for many years—until the survivor's oncologist gives the all-clear for the embryo to be transferred back to the woman. This way, a woman can experience the joys—and the less-than-stellar moments—of pregnancy and childbirth.

The risks with this procedure are twofold. First, in vitro fertilization (IVF) uses hormones to "ripen" a woman's eggs so that doctors can perhaps harvest more than one egg at a time. While working with multiple eggs increases the chances of success—just like your odds go up when you buy two lottery tickets rather than one—the catch here is that some breast cancers are hormonally responsive, and this process could stimulate breast cancer cells to grow, along with eggs.

Another concern is that, in order to do IVF, a patient must delay cancer treatment for about two weeks from the start of a period. Many cancers are slow-growing, so this delay isn't always a problem. But it can be dangerous for certain fast-growing cancers, such as acute leukemia.

On the other hand, it could work out nicely for women with breast cancer, at least those who have to heal from surgery before they are strong enough to start chemotherapy treatment. The IVF process might, as it did for Ilana, fit neatly into their schedules.

Successful egg retrieval, though, doesn't guarantee a baby. There's a level of attrition at each step, explains Lincoln. Not all eggs survive the thaw, though the figure is at about 90 percent. Then, not all eggs fertilize, whether they're fresh or frozen. Finally, not all embryos progress in order to be transferred. "I call it lottery tickets," says Lincoln. "You want to start with as many as you safely can" to improve your odds.

A side note to consider when freezing embryos is that, unlike eggs and sperm, embryos are not one-cell organisms. According to Lincoln, that means that doctors can safely extract a few cells from the outer cell mass of the embryo and test it for BRCA or other genetic mutations. It's impossible to test an egg or sperm without destroying it (and even if one is "clean," that doesn't mean any other egg or sperm cells in the batch are). Thus, before implanting the embryo, a cancer survivor can find out whether it carries a genetic mutation that could cause cancer.

It's an exciting advance—and one that is potentially controversial. But if you've been through the joys of cancer diagnosis and treatment, suggests Lincoln, you may appreciate the ability to know whether you're passing that propensity on to your child.

Egg Freezing. Women can also choose to freeze their eggs unfertilized, which might be an option for those who aren't in a committed relationship and don't have a sperm donor handy. The process of increasing egg production is the same. But instead of combining the eggs with sperm for fertilization, explains Haring, they are frozen immediately.

For years, fertility specialists have felt that freezing embryos was more effective than freezing eggs, but with advances in methods, that picture has changed. "We've certainly had more experience with freezing embryos," says Lincoln. "But the ability to freeze eggs has progressed so far with what we call vitrification of frozen eggs that now we're doing more and more with our egg donor bank," the onco-fertility specialist explains. "We think it works as well with our egg donor bank as fresh and we think it works as well in these patients also."

Lincoln points out that there are a couple of advantages to freezing eggs rather than embryos. First, the obvious: not everyone has a partner, and women might not want to use donor sperm if there's another option. Even if a woman does have a partner, it's hard to know what the future will bring, even for "regular" fertility patients, says Lincoln. Couples might get divorced, or a partner might die unexpectedly and the woman might decide to remarry, he suggests.

There are other concerns about an uncertain future. "Some couples don't want to create these embryos that they may not use sometime in the future," says Lincoln. "They are concerned about possibly having to dispose of them." There are fewer moral concerns associated with discarding frozen eggs than frozen embryos.

Freezing Ovarian Tissue. Some women choose to have parts of their ovaries surgically removed and frozen before treatment begins. Chances are, a piece of ovary—especially in a young woman—contains hundreds if not thousands of eggs. The advantage here is that freezing ovarian tissue doesn't affect hormone levels, which means it doesn't increase risk to hormone-receptor-positive breast cancer patients. "If a woman is at exceedingly high risk of losing ovarian function, we can do a laparoscopic surgery to remove one ovary and freeze it," says Susannah Copland, MD, of the Atlantic Reproductive Center.[5] Tissue is saved via cryopreservation.

The challenge with this approach is that these eggs are immature and must be grown in a lab, a process that is still in the experimental

---

5. Scott Huler, "A New Normal for Cancer Survivors," *Duke University Magazine*, Accessed December 4, 2013. http://www.dukehealth.org/health_library/health_articles/a_new_normal_for_cancer_survivors.

stage just now. Plus, doctors worry that returning a piece of ovary to the woman might inadvertently return a few cancer cells, too, which could, potentially, lead to recurrence.

Rachel went this route. After she was diagnosed with breast cancer in her early twenties, Rachel had chemotherapy and radiation as well as two mastectomies. She was luckier than Tito, though; her oncologist talked to her about fertility issues early on, before she even began treatment. "I'm not sure why he did," she says. "It's not like he had a lot of young cancer patients." And Rachel knew her own mind; she was sure she wanted to have children some day.

As a result, Rachel had her ovarian tissue frozen before she started treatment. "Just in case everything in there ended up getting destroyed by the chemo," she says. She considered freezing her embryos. But, as she explains, "I just didn't have that person in my life at that point that I felt like I wanted to freeze my eggs with."

Adapting the Treatment Protocol. A less common approach is to try to fiddle with the treatment protocol, if the onco docs determine that it is safe and appropriate, to make the treatment less likely to affect fertility.

For instance, some women receiving chemotherapy treatment can take a hormone that will put their ovaries into temporary menopause. The theory is that this will protect the ovaries from damage, but many infertility specialists doubt the approach's effectiveness, according to MD Anderson.[6] Another option is to surgically move the ovaries away from the radiation target field; according to MD Anderson, this results in a 50 percent chance that menstruation will resume after treatment. After you finish with cancer treatment, you

---

6. "Preserving Fertility Before Treatment," *MD Anderson Cancer Center*, accessed December 4, 2013, http://www.mdanderson.org/patient-and-cancer-information/cancer-information/cancer-topics/detection-and-diagnosis/preserving-fertility/index.html.

may need to have your ovaries repositioned again, or use IVF, in order to conceive.

Another option, depending on the situation, may be to remove just the uterus, instead of a full hysterectomy; this would allow the woman to retain reproductive capacity. Again, it is important to talk with your oncologists to determine the safest and most effective approach for your situation.

Age also plays a role in women's fertility, says Lincoln. "If we have a patient who's forty-four and wants to freeze her eggs, her risk of miscarriage is already at 50-plus percent," just because of her age, he explains. "We don't want to give out false hope and freeze a forty-five-year-old's eggs and say, 'You'll get pregnant, don't worry,' when that may really not be the case." As soon as the issue arises, speak with a fertility specialist. When you call for an appointment, make sure to mention that you're a cancer patient or survivor; as Ilana found out, it may facilitate scheduling.

Preserving Fertility in Men

The good news is that fertility preservation is generally cheaper, easier, and more effective for men. It's just a matter of collection through masturbation for a healthy post-pubescent male. Freezing sperm is nothing new; we've been doing it since the 1960s, according to Lincoln.

Ideally, several semen specimens should be cryo-preserved several times, every two or three days. This process could result in delaying treatment for a few days or maybe a week. The good part is that cryo-preserved sperm can be saved for years, sometimes even decades. It can be inseminated into a female partner or used with in vitro fertilization.

Sometimes, young men with cancer have poor sperm quality because of the disease, recent anesthesia, or stress. But even if there are only a few live sperm collected, the healthiest ones can still be captured, injected into a woman's harvested eggs, and prove effective. Recent developments with in vitro fertilization and ICSI (intracytoplasmic sperm injection) mean that even small numbers of sperm can result in pregnancy.

Saving Testicular Tissue. Another option for fertility preservation is saving testicular tissue, though it is an experimental procedure at this point.

Adapting the Treatment Protocol. Sometimes, oncologists can adapt the treatment protocol to preserve a man's fertility. For instance, if the cancer treatment involves radiation to the pelvis, radiation oncologists might be able to shield the testes, to preserve the man's fertility.

Similarly, men with low sperm counts or motility may find that their sperm improves after treatment is over. Again, though, this increased number and motility may not be enough to conceive without medical help. Physicians can examine a semen sample under a microscope to get a better sense of its fertility.

Children with Cancer

Adolescent angst is a rough time, but the advantage to having gone through it is that you can, at least, preserve your fertility if you have cancer. Fertility preservation is a lot more challenging in children. To put it bluntly, you can't collect eggs from an eight-year-old girl or sperm from a six-year-old boy. While it is possible to freeze ovarian or testicular tissue, both procedures are very much in the experimental stages. In fact, there have probably only been about twenty-five successful deliveries from ovarian or testicular tissue performed internationally, says Lincoln. Hopefully both processes will become easier and cheaper in the future. (Alternatively, I'd be happy with having cancer not hit the pre-pubescent crowd altogether.)

When Treatment Is Over

Fertility problems after cancer treatment aren't uncommon. *Fertility* is defined as the inability to conceive after one year of regular, unprotected intercourse. Nationwide, one in nine women and one in ten men ages fifteen through forty-four have fertility problems, according to the Centers for Disease Control and Prevention (CDC).[7] The stats are a little harsher for cancer survivors.

But that doesn't mean that everyone ends up with problems. Before assuming that your fertility is compromised, it's best to get tested and find out your fertility status. A fertility specialist can help with this. "There's no black and white answer to will you be able to get pregnant after whatever treatment," says Lincoln. It depends on what treatment you got and how old you were when you received it—as well as even more individual issues of personal fertility.

For women, the key time is about six months after treatment is over. You can have a complete hormonal screening, notes the Fertile Action website, to get a better sense of your fertility.[8] These tests, notes the nonprofit organization, could include

- Anti-mullerian hormone (AMH), which gives an indication of how many eggs you have left
- Antral follicle count, which approximates a count of eggs in your ovaries
- Follicle stimulating hormone (FSH), which determines how close you are to menopause
- Estradiol, which assesses the blood vessels and tissue of the endometrium
- Luteinizing hormone (LH), which triggers ovulation

Women who stop menstruating during treatment may get their periods back, though probably not right away. Often, it can take several months; for instance, I got my period back six months after finishing treatment. Even so, though, resumed menstruation does not guarantee regained fertility.

If there appears to be no ovarian function, women can get pregnant and carry it to term using donated eggs, called oocytes.

7. "Infertility FAQs," *Centers for Disease Control and Prevention*, accessed December 2, 2013, http://www.cdc.gov/Reproductivehealth/Infertility/#a.

8. http://www.fertileaction.org/learning-center/parenthood-after-cancer/overview/.

Some women use donors they know (relatives or friends), though most opt for anonymous donors. The donor is treated with fertility drugs to increase egg production. Once the eggs are retrieved, they can be fertilized with sperm from the survivor's partner, then placed into the survivor's uterus if feasible. Most IVF programs take patients up to age fifty. Women can also use donor eggs, according to OncoFertility Consortium.[9]

A man can get a semen analysis to determine whether there are sperm within his semen.[10] "Fertility Options." The OncoFertility Consortium. Accessed December 2, 2014. http://oncofertility. northwestern.edu/patients/fertility-preservation-options-nu Doctors determine sperm quality using at least these three "scores":

- Count: the number of sperm present. Typically there are at least twenty million sperm in each milliliter of semen.
- Motility: the percentage of sperm that are actively swimming around. Usually at least half of the sperm present should be moving.
- Morphology: the shape of the sperm. A relatively recent way to assess sperm, according to the American Society for Reproductive Medicine,[11] is that sperm must have a smooth, oval head; a well-defined cap; no visible defect of neck, midpiece, or tail; and no large fluid droplets in the sperm head. To be considered fertile, a man must have at least 4 percent normally shaped sperm.

It can take as long as a year—or even ten years—to return to normal levels of sperm production.

---

9. http://fertilitypreservation.northwestern.edu/decision-tree.

10. "Fertility Options," *The OncoFertility Consortium*, accessed December 2, 2013, http://oncofertility.northwestern.edu/patients/fertility-preservation-options-nu.

11. http://www.reproductivefacts.org/Sperm_Shape_Morphology_factsheet/.

Timing

Most people trying to get pregnant give it at least a year on their own before consulting a fertility specialist. But people who've been through chemotherapy or radiation are in a separate category, says Lincoln. They should probably figure out whether they need help sooner rather than later.

"Time is really critical," he says. "You don't want to lose two or three years wasting time with fertility treatments like IUI [intrauterine insertion—inserting sperm in a woman's uterus to facilitate fertilization] that aren't really going to help. Because now you're three years older than when you started." The biological clock ticks louder for cancer survivors, he suggests. "Basically, as soon as you're cleared to get pregnant from your oncologist, I would say that it's appropriate that you don't wait."

Pregnancy Post-Treatment

Before a survivor tries to get pregnant, though, there are a couple of things to consider. First, chemotherapy and radiation are very hard on various body parts, including the heart and lungs. Before a woman gets pregnant, therefore, she should have an echocardiogram to ensure that her heart is strong enough to handle pregnancy.

In addition, experts recommend waiting at least six months after treatment, because eggs that were maturing during treatment may be damaged by radiation or chemotherapy. Talk with your health-care provider, because the exact amount of time depends on the type and stage of cancer as well as the type of treatment received.

During this time, survivors should use birth control to avoid an unwanted pregnancy. Birth control pills, which use hormones to provide contraception, are generally not recommended if you've had breast cancer, according to Living Beyond Breast Cancer (LBCC), a national nonprofit advocacy organization.[12] Instead, stick with non-hormonal birth control methods, such as condoms, diaphragms, and non-hormonal IUDs (intra-uterine devices).

Women survivors are often thought to be in a more vulnerable place than their partners, says Katz, but in fact studies have shown that their partners often have higher emotional needs. In fact, studies show that women who believe their partner is emotionally invested in the relationship, and who have a positive first sexual experience after treatment, are likely to adjust well, Katz notes.

Stress doesn't help. And there's plenty of stress associated with trying to become pregnant. "The added stress of planning and timing can lead to decreased sexual desire, interest, and satisfaction," says Michael Krychman, MD, executive director of the Southern California Center for Sexual Health and sexual medicine gynecologist. "Women are also more likely to experience vaginal pain and dryness because the whole process can become stressful and regimented, affecting a couple's relationship during this time."

If a woman has had certain types of fertility sparing gynecologic surgery, such as a radical trachelectomy, or received radiation to the pelvic area, there is a greater chance of complication or miscarriage. Health-care providers consider these pregnancies high risk and, typically, monitor them accordingly. According to Fertile Hope, there is no reason to think that chemotherapy or radiation to other parts of the body would increase chances of miscarriage.[13]

---

12. Ann Honebrink, ed., "Early Menopause From Breast Cancer Treatment," *Living Beyond Breast Cancer*, last modified September 11, 2013, http://www.lbbc.org/Learn-About-Breast-Cancer/Early-Menopause-From-Breast-Cancer-Treatment.

13. "Pregnancy and Children After Cancer," *Fertile Hope*, accessed December 4, 2013, http://www.fertilehope.org/learn-more/cancer-and-fertility-info/pregnancy-and-children-after-cancer.cfm#q4.

Men should probably wait two to five years after treatment to try for pregnancy, according to cancer.net.[14] Researchers estimate that sperm damaged by chemo or radiation therapy should be repaired within two years.

There is no reason, given today's research, to worry about increased rates of birth defects. Breastfeeding also appears to be feasible unless, of course, your milk ducts were removed with a double mastectomy.

Cancer takes months of your life, your quality of life, and your sense of complacence. But with planning, determination, and luck, you can still have a family. And what better way is there to celebrate your "new life"?

Frequently Asked Questions

Q: Can cancer treatment cause infertility?

A: Certain types of surgery, chemotherapy, and radiation have the capacity to leave men and women infertile.

Q: Are there ways to test my fertility?

A: There are hormone tests to determine the fertility of both men and women.

Q: How can a woman prevent treatment-caused infertility?

A: Women can freeze their eggs or ovarian tissue, which may help with infertility.

Q: How can a man prevent treatment-caused infertility?

A: Men can freeze their sperm, which can help them with infertility issues.

Q: If I can, is it safe for me to become pregnant after cancer treatment?

A: Experts say that pregnancy is safe for cancer survivors and their babies.

---

14. "Having a Baby After Cancer," *Cancer.net*, January 1, 2013, http://www. cancer.net/coping/emotional-and-physical-matters/sexual-and-reproductive-health/having-baby-after-cancer-pregnancy.

Chapter 6

Other People's Reactions

Barbra was engaged to be married. She and her fiancé had known each other for three years and had plans to go to the Caribbean for Christmas. Then, in early December, she was diagnosed with breast cancer.

"He bailed when I told him," Barbra remembers. "It just blew me away. I thought, 'Oh my God, I'm such a bad judge of character.' I thought I knew this person." Barbara was stunned, not to mention feeling very, very alone.

"My breast surgeon told me from day one, because I told her what happened with my ex-boyfriend, 'This is the one time in your life where I'm telling you to be selfish. You come first; you have to come first. You're number one. You have to put all your energy into fighting this disease and beating it. And if people don't understand that, you can't be sitting there holding their hands, babysitting them to make them feel better. You're going through cancer; this is about you.'"

Tito, on the other hand, felt that everyone rallied around him when he was diagnosed with Hodgkin's disease at age seventeen. His family came to every chemotherapy treatment session, and his friends shaved their heads in solidarity, though perhaps that wasn't such a radical statement. "When a bunch of black teenagers shave their heads, it looks like fashion more than cancer," he explains.

People have all sorts of reactions to cancer. I have come to think of cancer as a sieve. Some people fall through the sieve and float down the drain. Just as important, if not more so, lots of people don't. It's those people who you know are the keepers—the people you know you can really count on. (Please note that I don't recommend a cancer diagnosis as a way to sort out your friends.)

For me, the most unnerving part of my first cancer experience concerned a friend from college. We had met in freshman English, became much closer in our senior year, and had been friends for a long time after graduation. She had visited me in Philadelphia, and I flew out to Oakland, California, when she was living there. When we both ended up living in New York City, we did lunch.

I met her for lunch shortly after I officially achieved complete hair loss—no more Bozo the Clown look. I decided, because she was an old friend and knew I was going through cancer treatment, she was bound to be supportive. I elected to be brave. I slathered my pate with sunscreen, put on lipstick (not exactly my style) and bright pink earrings (even less Beth-like), and headed out the door. I knew I was taking a chance, going out bold and bald. My spirits were buoyed when I got the thumbs-up from a few African American men who, incidentally, had foreheads that receded almost as far back as mine. I have to say, some of them looked pretty good.

I was early, having overcompensated for my chemo-paced stride, so I waited out front for my friend. When she approached, she literally took a step backward with a look of disgust on her face. Wow, I hadn't been expecting that. I apologized for surprising her.

We had an awkward and somewhat abbreviated lunch. I apologized, again, over the meal and in two subsequent emails.

It was months before I realized that I had nothing to apologize for. I had just come to lunch dressed as me. To be honest, I only figured it out after a gentle nudging from another friend.

I never heard from my lunch pal again.

On the flip side, the parents of my son's entire kindergarten first-grade class took me under its collective wing that year, including both people I knew well and those I had just met. When I think about it, I have a hard time coming up with something they *didn't* do for me. They accompanied me to doctor appointments and chemo treatments, brought us home-cooked meals, arranged for the most fabulous haircut I've ever had, offered conveniently timed play dates, you name it.

You never know what to expect, or who to expect it from. Or, at least, I didn't.

And, of course, some people have much more extreme experiences. Khit and Rachel both had boyfriends who broke up with them during treatment. And Barbra's fiancé dumped her when he found out about the diagnosis.

The good thing, though, about finishing treatment was that by that point, I knew who I could count on and who I couldn't. No more guesswork, no more treading gently, no more holding my breath. People had already passed—or flunked—the sieve test.

Mindy Greenstein had similar challenging experiences. She has an advantage, though. She can switch from her survivor hat to her psycho-oncologist hat and immediately analyze the situation. She describes people's responses as "breaking the daisy chain."

"We had a guy in group therapy who had been in the Korean War," she explains. "The guys in his troop felt that if they were all together in the same area, they'd be all right." If they were all together on the battlefield, they'd make it through the day. "That way, nobody would break the daisy chain."

It was all an illusion, of course. The guy admitted as much. On the battlefield, danger could hit the troops at any time, whether the guys were in one spot or spread apart over a larger area. But logic aside, the troops all felt safer if they were a unified group of Americans on foreign soil.

"That's sort of how I feel about cancer," Mindy explains. "It breaks the daisy chain for people who don't really want to be thinking about mortality." Cancer patients and survivors, just by our experiences, have raised a verboten topic for conversation. "This mortality thing that you brought into the space makes people nervous," Mindy says. It's just as true for kind, well-meaning people as for selfish ones, she adds.

"Even if you don't currently have cancer," Mindy adds, "people associate you with cancer. And then they want to dispel the anxiety that comes up for them because you had once broken the daisy chain."

People who couldn't handle my cancer diagnosis, then, weren't necessarily being unsupportive or mean—it could be that I had just scared the living daylights out of them.

If we can go through life perpetuating the myth of immortality, the faith in our own health and bodies, the daisy chain remains intact. But once someone reminds us that bad things *can* happen to good people, reminds us that life-threatening illnesses are more common than we'd like to believe, it shakes our confidence and we want to run away. We don't want to meet for lunch anymore.

The challenge, of course, is to keep that in mind when, for instance, a friend recoils from you.

The truth is that the number of people who did not fall through the sieve was numerically larger than the number who did. And these people were my true friends. Whether they sewed me hospital gowns, brought me food, or just treated me like "Beth" instead of "cancer girl," these are the people worth hanging onto.

Mindy agrees. "I found for the aftermath that the friendships that survived cancer were much more powerful, much stronger," Mindy says. "I had a real sense of gratitude for my friends that I hadn't had before, an appreciation of them."

Coping with Bad Reactions

The first decision, of course, is whether to deal with a situation at all, suggests Mindy. Think about what your needs are, what you want from the relationship. Is this an important person in your life? Often it is easier to hear thoughtless statements and questions from someone who is unimportant to you than it is to hear them from someone whose opinion really matters.

If the person isn't a good friend or family member, sometimes the simplest solution is just to avoid spending time with the person. A friend of mine, for instance, spent much of her time bemoaning how difficult it was for her to have a friend with cancer. We couldn't have a single conversation on any other topic—even my comments about the hot weather were trumped by the sort of back-handed sympathy that really bothered me. I didn't want to spend my time cheering her up, so I decided, instead, to spend less time with her altogether.

If, on the other hand, the person who is hurting your feelings is important to you, if it is someone you genuinely care about, that is a different story. "It can be hard to remember that when people are being jerks to us that they're dealing with their fears, whether they know it or not," says Mindy. You are, after all, sort of forcing them to think about their own mortality every time they ask how you are feeling.

In those cases, it is in your best interests to help the person to help you. Often, the person is really trying his or her best. As Mindy says, "People, they often don't know what to say. They might say something terrible and an hour later, they're thinking, oh my God, I shouldn't have said that to her. They're going through a process, too."

The best way, the gentlest way, to help your friend, suggests Mindy, is to start by pointing out something she does that is helpful, followed by a comment that feels a little less helpful. Taking a clue from Mary Poppins, it's a matter of sugar-coating the critique while helping your pal learn how to be a better friend in a difficult situation.

"You want to let them know in as easy a way as possible," says Mindy. "You can say, when you said X, it was really, really helpful for me. When you said Y, it made me realize that it's better for me not to hear things like that," she suggests. "So if you can point out something that's helpful along with something that's unhelpful, the other person might respond better."

Sometimes, you are close enough to the person that you can be even more explicit with your request, says Mindy. "With my mother, for instance, there are things that I tell her she's not allowed to say to me. For instance, she isn't allowed to cry in front of me."

Mindy made that quite clear soon after her diagnosis. "I told her, 'If you're going to cry, I'm hanging up. You can cry to Daddy, you can cry to my brother, but don't cry to me.'" Again, though, this has a lot to do with the nature of the relationship before cancer. A casual acquaintance, for instance, might not take well to receiving this sort of direction.

Sometimes, no matter how difficult the comments, it is easier to listen to hurtful statements than to deal with the response—because everything you say has ripple effects. "It's a complicated balancing act of deciding what makes you feel worse—hearing the statement or dealing with the consequences of saying something" says Mindy. In these cases, probably the easiest approach is to try to remember that, chances are, the person means well but just can't express her concern in a helpful manner.

What I learned, ultimately, from dealing with other people after cancer, is that I have control over how I react to what they say. I can decide to ignore the comments, ignore the person, or try to redirect the way the person talks with me. In fact, sometimes just knowing that I get to make a decision about the situation helps me field repeated awkward comments without crying or yelling or ruining my (or the other person's) day.

"I hear this from survivors a lot, that when treatment is over, people look at you as being victorious and they expect you to get back and show up for life," says Elissa. "They kind of congratulate you. And I'm like, 'I'm not sure I did anything that's very victorious.'"

Donna agrees. "The 'you're so strong' thing is condescending and patronizing," she says. She finds she avoids that sort of "cheerleader."

I have found that the best thing to do when people make well-meaning yet hurtful comments is to call up a member of the cancer club and kvetch. I try not to take it out on the well-meaning friend or acquaintance. But if I don't tell someone about it, it drives me crazy. Fortunately, whoever I've ever called with this complaint has always had a comparable story. We usually have a lovely kvetch-sharing chat.

Short Attention Span

The other challenge of being a survivor is that people have short attention spans. They're ready for you to be done with cancer and "back to normal," whatever that means. After all, it's hard work to deal with the physical limitations that come along with cancer treatment. It's annoying to have to help out and to pick up the slack.

In Elissa's case, as her hair started to grow in, she was expected back at work and the car pool. "I was like walking and standing and they're like, OK, it's time to start driving the car pool again, it's time to start doing the grocery shopping, it's time to start making your own meals," Elissa says.

Sometimes that is just fine.

Donna, for instance, wanted to pick up where she left off. She doesn't agree with the idea of "pulling life together again." She explains, "I'm just continuing what I'm doing. . . . This is what's now, and what's tomorrow will be different. . . . I just go along a continuous road," she says. "I don't feel like I was pulling myself together. Life after cancer is pretty much the same as before."

Others, though (myself included), feel different after treatment, and need some time to sort out what happened. Elissa, too, falls into this category. "I felt like I really needed to grieve and to feel like, almost like I was in mourning for a while after cancer," she says.

"I talk to patients a lot about this. It's a process, it's a marathon, not a sprint," Elissa explains. "You're going to have good days and bad days, and you have to be patient with yourself. Which is a lot easier for me to say than to follow," she adds. "I'm definitely not a very patient person. But I think that for most patients it gets better with time. It's OK to be upset and sad and worried for a while—even as long as a year, as long as it's not interfering with your day-to-day life."

Rachel found that people were great when she was coping with breast cancer, but when she had a prophylactic mastectomy a few years later, it was a different story. "Because it wasn't a cancer diagnosis, because it wasn't life threatening and it was a choice of mine, a lot of friends weren't really supportive," she remembers.

Rachel remembers one friend with whom she'd had a "really silly argument." "She didn't talk to me for two months—and those two months were the two months I was recovering from my mastectomy," Rachel says. It was the time when she really needed a friend. "It was so odd that people treated this mastectomy so much differently than the first one. I didn't have the same support; I didn't have people constantly asking how I was and coming over to visit and dropping things off," she remembers.

She still needed the concern. "I was still in that emotional place where I needed that support from my friends and family," says Rachel. "You think they're going to have your back again, like they did before." But they just weren't there for her.

The first time around, Rachel's confidence came from her friends' support and caring. "The fact that it wasn't there this time around," she says, "meant that I had to kind of do it for myself. I had to find things for myself that would give me confidence." In the long run, Rachel says that the experience, while painful, has been useful for her.

"I think that learning to rely more on myself for my happiness and confidence and looking at the real friends I had in my life actually made me a lot stronger," she says. "It took a lot of hard work, but I'm glad that I was able to turn this into a positive experience. Rather than something that's ruined my life, it's actually something that's made it better. I probably lost three or four friends on my cancer journey. But the ones who remain are special." Plus, she's added a few more friends along the way.

Not all of Rachel's friends disappeared. "I realized that beforehand, my friendships were based around the fact that we would go out all the time—we would do something, go get drunk, have stupid times," she says. "Basically like young twenties kinds of things." But after treatment, Rachel wasn't interested in those sorts of activities. "I still, to this day, don't go out to drink and do the same things that I did when I was younger," says the twenty-seven-year-old. Now she's more likely to hang out and talk, or see a movie. "It's sort of a deeper connection, rather than just a surface young twenties thing to do. I don't like going out and getting drunk and being hungover—it reminds me of chemo."

Rachel feels like a different person now. "I guess all in all, the whole cancer treatment taught me to look deeper into people rather than the surface stuff," she says, "in all sorts of relationships." She has changed the way she relates to her friends. "I definitely express my feelings a little bit more than before. It's cheesy sometimes. I tell my friends how much I appreciate them and how much I love them." And it's all to the good, in Rachel's mind. "I think it's brought me a lot closer to a lot of friends, because we've made that deeper connection. Everything's different. And so much better. Its deeper and better and more fulfilling," she says.

Again, it's a matter of understanding how you're reacting to surviving cancer, what you want and need from the people around you, and how to enable them to help you. Most people mean well; try to remember that. I find, though, that it helps to have an idea of what to expect. You might still be disappointed, but you're less likely to be taken by surprise.

Perhaps most important, it helps to find a fellow survivor, or two, who can sympathize with you when it comes to dealing with non-cancer civilians. Sometimes talking with another survivor is the best way to deal with other people who haven't had their own cancer journey.

Frequently Asked Questions

Q: Why do people make thoughtless remarks to cancer survivors?

A: Often, when people see someone who has faced down a life-threatening illness, they feel scared, as it reminds them of their own mortality. They may not even be aware of their emotional response—or of how it sounds to you. Usually, they mean well, but the compassion doesn't always come across that way.

Q: Do I have to continue to talk with people who hurt my feelings every time we chat?

A: No, the cancer survivor's needs come first; your needs come first. The key is to think through whether you want to say something and what the consequences may be.

Q: How do I tell my friend that he or she is upsetting me? I don't want to hurt his or her feelings.

A: Usually the gentlest way to critique someone is to start out by praising something he or she does that is kind or helpful. Then, suggest that not all of his or her comments are equally supportive and suggest an alternative that would help you feel better. People often respond well to well-intended suggestions made in a kind manner.

Section 2

Career Introduction

A cancer diagnosis can be a wake-up call, nudging people to rethink their career choices and work-life balance. After all, we spend a good chunk of our time and energy on the job, and who wants to be miserable for forty-plus hours a week? Survivors who have had to take time off work for treatment have probably had time to really think through their life and work choices. It's a chance to view your livelihoods with fresh eyes.

Sometimes survivors realize they're exactly where they want to be professionally. But sometimes those fresh eyes are cynical ones.

Unfortunately, figuring out what you want to do doesn't necessarily mean you're able to do it. Lots of survivors, unfortunately, run into difficulties in the work force, for all sorts of reasons. Researchers in Amsterdam found that cancer survivors have a higher level of unemployment than the rest of the population. It can be tougher on some than on others. Survivors of breast, cervical, endometrial, ovarian, and gastrointestinal cancer are more likely than others to be unemployed. And, oddly, chances are that a certain amount of that has to do with the work environment in the United States; European cancer survivors, the study reports, do much better in the workforce than American ones.[1]

As a rule, cancer survivors don't work as much after cancer treatment as they did before, statistically speaking. Cancer survivors are likely to work two to four fewer hours a week, even as much as two to six years after diagnosis.[2]

That sounds like a good thing, but most of the difference stems from people who had recurrences or developed new cancers. "We don't know if the reductions we observed are voluntary, perhaps reflecting people's changing priorities in the face of a serious illness, or if they are the result of forces beyond their control, such as employment discrimination or inadequate workplace accommodations," said John Moran, PhD, associate professor of health policy and administration in the College of Health and Human Development at Pennsylvania State University, who headed up the study.

Most survivors, though, don't think this is the ideal situation. Many want to work as much after treatment as before.

First of all, there's that minor incentive of needing to pay the rent and stock the refrigerator. But beyond that, most cancer survivors want to return to normal as possible and feel productive—though, of course, lots of people do want to re-jigger their work-life balance.

This book is not meant to take the place of the many excellent volumes out there on job searches. It just focuses on those special challenges specific to people who've survived cancer.

---

1. de Boer et al., "Cancer Survivors and Unemployment: A Meta-Analysis and Meta-Regression," *Health Services Research* 43 (2008): 193–210.

2. Short et al., "Long-Term Effects of Cancer Survivorship on the Employment of Older Workers," *National Center for Biotechnology Information* 43 (2008): 193–210. doi: 10.1111/j.1475-6773.2007.00752.x.

Chapter 7

Returning to the Job

When she was diagnosed with stage-four inflammatory breast cancer, Donna craved normalcy. She wanted her "old" life back, both personally and professionally. She enjoyed her work as an English-as-a-Second-Language (ESL) teacher in New York City. Her students really kept her on her toes, and Donna continued teaching throughout chemotherapy and radiation treatment.

But the mastectomy was another story; she couldn't just work through that. It was major surgery, and Donna needed a little time to rest and recoup afterward. Thankfully, the Family Medical Leave Act (FMLA) enabled her to take some time off while keeping her health insurance and job. (For more information on the law, see Chapter 9: Legal Issues.)

As soon as Donna started feeling better, she was eager to get back to the classroom. She missed her students, her colleagues, and the sense of accomplishment she got from helping immigrants and international students get a handle on the subtleties of the English language. She didn't want to sit home anymore.

"I like my job, and it feels good to be of service," Donna says. "I was glad I had to get up and out. Taking time off wouldn't have served me," she says. "I wanted to keep going; I didn't want to become too self-absorbed."

"I especially like my job when people give it back, when the energy system works both ways, when it's not only the teacher expending energy and the student sitting it out," Donna says. She's also fond of the people she works with. "My colleagues are great, and I generally like most of the students. When I came back, people said, 'Yeah, you're back!'" In fact, these days, because of her fatigue, most of Donna's social life comes from her interactions with the other teachers and with her students.

Fortunately for Donna, the logistics of taking time off and of returning to her job were pretty simple. The classes she teaches are offered in bite-sized chunks of six weeks each, so Donna finished up one term, had surgery, took it easy for a bit, and came back just in time to take on a full complement of courses. Her boss was fine with it, and no one was inconvenienced. No colleague had to fumble around with unfamiliar lesson plans, and no students got lost in the shuffle, thanks to an organized and compassionate supervisor. And a couple of teachers who could use some extra income got a little more in their take-home pay.

Donna was very lucky.

Unfortunately, not everybody has such good feelings about returning to work post-treatment, says Julie Jansen, career coach and author of *I Don't Know What I Want But I Know It's Not This: A Step-by-Step Guide to Finding Gratifying Work*. She has worked with hundreds of men and women, helping them sort out these issues.

"The majority of people are nervous, scared, fearful, and worried" when they think about going back to their jobs after finishing treatment, says Jansen. "There might be a little bit of excitement, there might be a little bit of positive anticipation. But I think, for the most part, people are very nervous," she adds.

It makes sense when you think about it. Lots of things have changed for someone who's been through cancer. "They're different people now, in many ways," says Jansen. "They worry: How are people going to view me? Am I going to be able to do my job? Will I want to do my job? Will people treat me differently?"

It's hard to know exactly what to expect, and it's difficult to prepare when you don't know what you're getting ready for. So it's best to walk in knowing that there may well be surprises.

Managing the Work

Probably the two biggest challenges when it comes to returning to a job following cancer treatment are handling the work itself and managing your relationships with supervisors, colleagues, and clients, Jansen says.

It helps to do some serious thinking about what to expect before you go back. Remember, you're not exactly the same person you were when you received the diagnosis. Your body has been fighting a major battle using extremely powerful weaponry. Unfortunately, those weapons take a toll on the body's healthy cells along with the cancerous ones.

Even though you've won the battle now, you may not have quite the strength, stamina, or perseverance you had before. Your short-term memory and ability to multi-task may be compromised, thanks to chemobrain, the thinking and memory problems that often stem from chemotherapy. You may have all kinds of weird side effects, from leg pains to ongoing nausea, and from loss of feeling in your fingers and toes (neuropathy) to elevated cholesterol.

Some challenges are cancer-specific. Breast cancer survivors, for instance, might face lymphedema, which can make it hard to move your arm. You might also be a little less sure of yourself; your body failed you, so it's hard to be as confident as you used to be. Maybe you're right; right after treatment, survivors are often more susceptible to infection.

That was Sherry's story. When she was diagnosed with ovarian and endometrial cancer, Sherry had been a high-level administrator in Washington, DC–based nonprofit organizations devoted to Native American issues. She managed programs and staff. Shortly after she finished surgery and started chemotherapy, she went back to the office. Everyone was glad to see her, supervisors and colleagues alike. But shortly after she returned, Sherry ended up in the hospital for a week, because of an infection that was difficult to treat.

"At that point," Sherry says, "I decided not to go back to work."

Fortunately, Sherry worked for an organization that was particularly supportive. Plus, she'd been there a long time and had strong connections with everyone in the office. "I had worked for them for about sixteen or seventeen years at that point," she explains. "I realized I was really pushing it, trying to go back to work so quickly," she says.

Through a combination of short-term disability, long-term disability, and an unusually generous employer, Sherry was able to take what the office called a "sabbatical." Not that lying in bed to recuperate from cancer treatment is exactly the typical sabbatical activity. Sherry also did a little writing and other work from home during this time.

Alas, Sherry's post-treatment infection isn't so unusual. I know that after my mastectomy, I had a hospital-related infection—and then a bad reaction to the medicines I was prescribed to treat it. According to the Institute of Medicine, about one in five cancer survivors will experience some sort of cancer-related work limitations up to five years after they finish treatment. Hopefully these people won't have problems convincing their employers to make the necessary accommodations (see Chapter 10: Legal Issues for more details on legal rights in the workplace).

Making Changes at Work

Some people find that when they get back to the office, they have to make some changes to function well. Maybe they need certain files moved to a lower cabinet drawer, for instance, or access to a nearby printer.

Donna was lucky. She encountered no difficulties in the classroom. Her voice was fine, and her teaching style had long encompassed a combination of sitting and standing. She just found herself doing a little more of the former, a little less of the latter. Luckily, she hasn't experienced any lymphedema (at least thus far), so she can easily gesture and write on the blackboard. "That was my biggest fear," she explains. "It would have been harder to go back to the classroom if I had lymphedema."

Even without lymphedema, though, Donna wasn't feeling 100 percent when she returned to work. That's not surprising for someone who'd been through surgery, chemotherapy treatment, and radiation. So, to manage her workload, she made a few changes to her work life.

As soon as she was diagnosed, Donna dropped some extra weekend hours she had been working. "I let go of Sundays," she explains. "Normal full-time at the school is thirty hours a week. Monday to Thursday, four hours in the morning and four hours at night." Her supervisor found a replacement teacher for the extra time, allowing Donna to switch to "just" full-time work. That way, she had chemo on Friday morning and had the rest of the day, along with Saturday and Sunday, to recuperate. "I needed the rest," says Donna. "I didn't have anything to prove."

Donna benefits from the unconventional teaching schedule at her school. Because classes are held in the mornings and evenings, Donna gets time to rest midway through each day. "When I was in chemo, I kept promising myself, 'Five hours and you'll be back home for a nap,'" she remembers. It worked then, and, even these days, a year after finishing treatment, a nap is sometimes an enticing option.

Donna plans to stick with that schedule. "I wasn't hired to work on Sundays in the first place," she says. "It's really delicious to have a few days where I lay around." Making use of her time off, Donna is becoming somewhat of an authority on *Law and Order* and *Gossip Girl*. "I call it enforced stillness."

Donna made one other change to her work life. She switched work locations for the evening classes. The school where she works has several sites in the area, but only one is within walking distance of Donna's home; she had been working at a location that required a thirty-minute bus ride.

While she was in radiation treatment, Donna asked her supervisor if she could teach at the closer location in the evenings. That way she'd only have to make the longer commute once a day. "I figured if there was ever a time to really request something, it was then."

Whether Donna and her supervisor realized it or not, they were following the law. Being proactive is key. The Americans with Disabilities Act (ADA) requires people to anticipate issues rather than wait until problems crop up. In fact, if someone gets a poor review because of cancer-related challenges, that black mark stays on her permanent record, even if the company makes a modification that addresses the concern later on. If Donna had waited until she'd been late to class a couple of times, for instance, she would have sullied her work performance record, even if she was able to change locations a few weeks into the term. By changing her evening classroom site before she got too exhausted, before her fatigue affected her work, Donna avoided that situation.

Donna was also lucky about her supervisor, who sympathized with the request and asked some of the staff members if they would be willing to switch with Donna. One woman volunteered. "She was happy to do it. She was extremely supportive of me, and she had a car, so the commute wasn't as hard for her," says Donna.

The switch in work locations is permanent. So, now, when the weather is nice, Donna gets a walk in every day she works, strolling about a mile to and from class. That exercise can be helpful in trying to prevent recurrence (for more information on the benefits of exercise, see Chapter 12: Exercise).

Donna made one other change in her life, a change that has nothing to do with the school, her supervisor, colleagues, or students. It's internal. She's learning to give herself a break. "It is tiring, teaching sixteen classes a week," she says. "That's a reality for anybody—sixteen classes is a lot of classes." She thinks about college teachers who often have a quarter of that load. Or less. "Some days I phone in the job, and other days I'm super prepared," says Donna, downplaying her skills. "But that's kind of normal for most people." Donna tries hard to remember that everyone has good days and bad, whether they're in treatment or not, whether they've had cancer or not. "A job always has its ups and downs, but ultimately I like my work, and I like to keep learning."

Managing the Relationships

The other challenge of returning to your old job is managing the relationships with your supervisor, colleagues, and clients. That's always a part of work, but it can be a particularly worrisome task when you're coming back to the office after medical leave.

Donna had no trouble talking to her immediate supervisor about the accommodations she needed to keep doing her job. They had a good relationship, and Donna's boss was eager to help. That's great news for Donna, but it's not always the case.

Donna also had an easy time sharing her situation with everyone else at the school, from colleagues to students. She'd made the decision early on that she was going to be totally up front about her cancer. She found that everyone was very understanding and supportive. Some people even told her that they considered her a hero, though she wasn't thrilled by that comment. "I don't know what that was about," Donna says. "I just did what I had to do."

It was a good thing that Donna shared her diagnosis and treatment with her employer. She's the kind of person who would have had a difficult time keeping it secret. "It was obvious I was sick," she says, though she always wore a hat to work to cover her bald head. She just wasn't her old self.

"I have nice colleagues, and we can shoot the breeze," she says. Some of the students knew what was going on, too, offering reassurance. But not everyone was aware that Donna had cancer. One student who didn't know said, "She's crazy; she cut off all her hair," Donna remembers, laughing.

Unfortunately, not everyone feels that's a safe approach to take at the job. Julie, for instance, had a part-time gig managing an academic journal. Given how her boss had reacted to other people's situations, Julie figured discretion was the way to go.

She worked mostly from home, and was in a managerial role, so she juggled the deadlines to avoid working while she was in the intensive care unit. Thanks to the magic of cell phones, no one knew that she was working with the copyeditor and authors wearing a hospital gown instead of jeans. "I know my boss would have fired me if he had known I had cancer," she says. "So I picked the easy way out: I never told him."

Even people who work in an office all the time can be coy with their health information, notes Jansen. "We see a wide range from people who absolutely share nothing and they just soldier forward to people who are completely an open book," Jansen says.

When you think about it, that range of approaches is always the case. Cancer or no cancer, there are always some people who are familiar with the details about your lousy date on Friday night and others who don't know anything more personal about you than your opinion on the break room coffee. "You don't treat every single person in your life the same way, nor would you do it in this situation," Jansen notes. "You're going to communicate differently with each person, just as if you were healthy."

The key to managing relationships when you come back after cancer treatment, says Jansen, is to think it through in advance, not just react to comments as they're thrown your way. Decide how you're going to approach it; don't just wing it.

"When most people go to work, they don't spend a lot of time thinking about their relationships, which I believe is a mistake," Jansen says. Most people focus on finalizing the details of the ad campaign, fiscal report, or other project. But Jansen thinks we should all put energy into maintaining our relationships with supervisors and colleagues. Not just when there are extenuating situations, but all the time. "When you've been put into this situation where you've been ill, then you really *have* to think about your relationships and you *have* to manage them—and manage communication," she reiterates.

Why bother with office politics? Don't you have enough to deal with between handling the fatigue and other symptoms, figuring out the company's latest software program, and deciphering the handwritten notes from the guy who did part of your job while you were out?

Well, as Jansen explains, when you come back after a medical leave of absence, "the cards are stacked against you. People are thinking you're weak or still sick or can't carry your part of the work load." Some people may start out thinking you're fine, she observes. "But if there's any slippage, if there's any sign of weakness, no matter what," people chalk it up to cancer and assume that you just can't do the job anymore.

"There's going to be a sign of weakness for anybody, no matter what—cancer or no cancer," says Jansen. That's true even for someone who feels completely strong and healthy, which is rather rare under these circumstances. "I don't know anybody who's been through cancer who feels 100 percent when they finish treatment," says Jansen. Whether there's a typo in your memo, you forget about a meeting, or you just can't remember where they keep the extra ballpoint pens—that's it. "When in doubt, people defer to the negative," warns Jansen.

Most people, though, aren't malicious. Some will be supportive—pleased to see you back in the office and eager to help however they can. Others will worry that you will fall behind and their workload will increase. They may not intend to make your life more difficult; they just don't want any more demands on theirs.

Part of the challenge to managing work relationships is that you don't *really* know what people are thinking and saying about you. (Anyone who thinks that their workplace is free of politics, well, I'd love to work in your office. A 2012 Robert Half study found that 54 percent of office workers admit to gossiping or spreading rumors about office politics.[1] And those are just the people who admit their feelings to a polltaker.)

"People aren't necessarily honest about what they're thinking or feeling about you," says Jansen. "Either they like you and they don't want to hurt your feelings, or maybe they're a little bit more self-centered about their situation, about getting the work done." They may say everything is fine while they are mentally composing a complaining email to their friend—or boss.

"Here's the problem with anything having to do with people," says Jansen. "It's not a science—it's an art." So, to deal with people, you need to be a bit of an artist, dealing in subtleties.

Of course, there's also the question of whether you are able—or willing—to fall back into all your old work patterns. Are you still prepared (or able) to work until eight o'clock at night most days of the week? Are you still patient enough to sit through interminable and unproductive meeting after interminable and unproductive meeting? Are you OK with hearing people kvetch about their twenty-four-hour flu (compared with six months of chemo-induced nausea), lousy haircut (versus complete hair loss), or fatigue because of a late night (as opposed to months of being bone-tired)?

---

1. "Psst . . . Have You Heard the News about Office Politics?" *Robert Half International*, Aug. 23, 2012, http://rhfa.mediaroom.com/2012-08-23-Psst-...-Have-You-Heard-The-News-About-Office-Politics.

Donna has found that she has become much less patient with negative attitudes since she faced down cancer. Most of us survivors are in line right behind her. Many people who've been faced with cancer find that they want to adjust the role that work plays in their lives, what people call work-life balance. Donna, for instance, decided to stick with a full-time course load rather than add a weekend course to her responsibilities. Most people—more than two-thirds (67 percent), according to a survey by the nonprofit group Cancer and Careers[2]—experience some challenges navigating this delicate balance.

Who to Talk to—Does Size Matter?

Part of managing your work relationships involves knowing who to talk to about what. If you work at a small company, there's no question: you have to talk to your supervisor about when you return to work and any reasonable accommodations you might need. There's no other option. If you're at a larger firm, though, should you go to your supervisor or to the human resources department to make arrangements?

Jensen explains that company culture is more important than size, while it is true that big companies are more likely than smaller ones to have a Human Resources department. HR is probably the corporate expert on the legal niceties of taking time off and making accommodations to the work environment. Sometimes that may be the way to go.

"People often pick HR if they are hoping to reveal only as much about their health situation as necessary to avail themselves of company policies or legal protection," says Rebecca Nellis, vice

2. "Newly Released Survey Reveals the Majority of Cancer Patients and Survivors Want to Continue Working," *PRNewswire*, March 5, 2013, www.prnewswire. com/news-releases/newly-released-survey-reveals-the-majority-of-cancer-patients-and-survivors-want-to-continue-working-195252221.html.

president, programs and strategy of the nonprofit organization Cancer and Careers. "Beyond company policy, HR often has knowledge of how other people with cancer or serious medical issues managed work and can provide some helpful insights and ideas," she adds.

But you may have a really good relationship with your supervisor, like Donna does. Donna arranged everything through her supervisor without involving HR at all. That's not so unusual, says Jansen. Nelllis agrees. Sometimes "a manager or supervisor is the person they feel most comfortable talking to, and often they can be great sources of support as well as advocates within the company." Sometimes, even when there is an HR department, it can be best to discuss everything directly with your manager. It's very situational—there's no one-size-fits-all answer.

"There are some smaller companies where everybody's really tight, and everybody has a great relationship, and they're very understanding," says Jensen. "And then there are other smaller environments that are very toxic." So, here, like with many things survivorship-related, you have to play it by ear.

Balancing on the Work-Life Seesaw

The first thing I think of when I hear the term work-life balance is a playground seesaw. I remember how much fun it can be when both people work together—when you push off the sand with your feet and soar through the air, accompanied by the sounds of your and your partner's giggles. For some reason, all the seesaws I remember sat in large sandboxes. Eventually, though, someone's mom calls out that it is time to go home, and, if it's not *your* mom, you probably end up with your ass in the sand.

Balancing work with the rest of your life, and balancing the work relationships necessary, can be just as, well, up and down—alternately glorious and precarious, with a distinct possibility of ending up with sand down your pants.

Usually when people want something different, it's a change in the work-life balance, says Jansen. Some people go back to their old jobs, then realize that it isn't working out. The cancer experience, says Jansen, makes people sit up and take notice. "Who cares how many legal briefs I write, or who cares how many advertising campaigns I put together, or who cares how many media placements I've gotten for someone, or how many projects I've managed?" says Jansen. "It doesn't seem to matter anymore. It isn't meaningful anymore."

"You find people on every part of the spectrum. Some people want everything to be completely different than it was before they had cancer," says Jansen. "Some people just crave normalcy—they just want to get back to what their normal was before they got their diagnosis," says Jansen. "And then they get there, and they're in shock because they realize that they don't want it to be the same." They think they want exactly what they had—until they show up at the job and realize that they don't.

The key is to talk with your company before you head back to work. "You can't just decide to go home at five o'clock," says Jensen. "You need to talk with your manager about that." There's really no way around it. "Either you go in to your manager and say, 'I can't work until eight o'clock, so can we make some concessions," says Jensen, or you work until eight o'clock and feel resentful and tired.

I think about the way Donna changed her approach to work. She gave herself permission to work at 97 percent or 98 percent every so often, not charging ahead 110 percent every single day. Sometimes just being kind to yourself can make a big difference in how you view your work, in the internal work-life balance.

The truth of the matter, if you look at the research, is that most survivors end up working with a similar work-life balance as they had before their cancer journey. They often ease into it, though. A Swedish study found that three out of four women treated for breast cancer (75 percent) had returned to their pre-diagnosis work schedule by sixteen months after they returned to work. Only about one in seven women actually cut her work hours, but that usually had more to do with some treatment-related work limitation than anything else.[3]

But you can be that one in seven, if it suits your needs and the needs of your employer. And if you arrange it in advance.

Contingency Planning

Donna was lucky; for her, going back to work was a smooth process. She has a good reputation at the school, and people were glad to see her back. Her students like her; her colleagues like her. She had a good handle on the things she wanted to remain the same (responsibilities and colleagues) and those she wanted to change (location and number of hours). But, says Jansen, not everyone is so lucky.

"When you think about contingency planning, you shouldn't approach it from a negative standpoint—if I go back, it's not going to work out," Jansen says. "But at the same time, you want to be thinking about a contingency plan," she cautions. "Don't wait until you get there and discover that there's a problem." If you expect to drive down a well-paved road and then hit an icy patch, in other words, you could end up scrambling for a solution. Best to pull out those snow tires in advance.

Concrete Steps: Preparing to Return

OK, you've decided it. You're ready to go back to your job. You've thought long and hard, and you're confident you can do it. But it's not quite as simple as dressing the part and grabbing your commuter pass.

You don't have to gun your motor and break the speed limit on day one. Assess how you feel. Do you want to start out part-time, or are you ready to plunge back into full-time work? Are there times of day that work better than others for you? Donna was lucky; her

---

3. Høyer et al., "Change in Working Time in a Population-Based Cohort of Patients With Breast Cancer," *Journal of Clinical Oncology* (2012), doi:10.1200/ JCO.2011.41.4375.

class schedule had an afternoon break built into it. She could always promise herself an afternoon nap. I worked as a freelance writer and editor from my living room; that lovely, inviting bed was never more than a few steps away. But many office jobs require people to work for eight (or more) hours straight—and in professional attire, no less. Are you up to it?

Think about whatever medications you're taking. Do they have any weird side effects that might get in your way? Can you drive to work? Do you have the energy to stand up all day? Will you be able to stay alert during marathon meetings (well, at least as alert as everyone else)? Will you be able to be on your feet all day, without taking periodic rests? (Alternately, can you build those rests into your workday without annoying colleagues and supervisors?)

If you're not sure you're quite ready, there might be a therapist in your area who can help talk you through your options. Or there might be a support group of other survivors who are also re-entering the workforce. It's nice not to have to go it alone.

Ergonomics

When you're thinking about preparing to go back to work and assessing your working conditions, it's probably useful to remember ergonomics. I know that I always just sort of coped with having shorter-than-average legs at a normal-person-sized desk for years, but after treatment, I found it really bugged me. And you may as well ask for all the changes you need at one time.

Ergonomics are always important, even if you're in perfect health, according to the Occupational Safety and Health Administration (OSHA), which is part of the U.S. Department of Labor. Poor ergonomics can cause tendinitis, muscle strain, lower back pain, and carpal tunnel syndrome. The OSHA website offers specific recommendations for a wide variety of professions, but we'll just take a look at two common concerns here: desk workers and health-care employees.

Sitting at a desk seems like a safe place to be. After all, you're not exactly digging in a coal mine, hanging off a skyscraper cleaning windows, or parachuting into enemy territory. But it's still good to keep your body in a neutral position, to reduce stress and strain. OSHA recommends keeping your

- Hands, wrists, and forearms straight and parallel to the floor.
- Head level, or bent slightly forward so that it is in line with the torso.
- Shoulders relaxed, with your upper arms at your sides.
- Elbows close to the body and bent at about ninety degrees to 120 degrees.
- Feet sitting flat on the floor. If you can't adjust your desk height, consider using a footrest.
- Back fully supported, with appropriate support when sitting vertical or leaning back slightly. A good chair is critical.
- Thighs and hips supported by a well-padded seat and situated parallel to the floor.
- Knees in line with the hips, feet slightly forward.[4]

When it comes to the health-care arena, lifting patients is a big challenge for nurses and nursing assistants trying to take good care of their backs and legs. OSHA makes the following recommendations:

- Don't transfer people if you're feeling at all off balance.
- Lift loads close to your body.
- Never lift alone, especially if the patient has fallen. Try to use mechanical assistance, or at least another health-care professional.
- Limit the number of lifts you do each day.
- Avoid lifting when your spine is rotated.

---

4. "Good Working Positions," *U.S. Department of Labor*, accessed December 4, 2013, https://www.osha.gov/SLTC/etools/computerworkstations/positions.html.

- Use mechanical assistance whenever possible—and take advantage of all training on the subject. The easiest way to avoid injuring your back is to limit how you use it.[5]

While this may seem like a lot to ask from your employer, it's probably easiest to ask all at once. Plus, coming out of treatment, you're a little more fragile now than you were before diagnosis. Take care of yourself and encourage your employer to do the same.

Getting Your Feet Wet

Some people like to jump into a cold pool and dunk their head under water all at once, to get the shock over with. Other people start by dipping their toes in and adjusting to the temperature bit by bit.

When it comes to going back to work after cancer treatment, lots of people are toe dippers. There are many ways you can prepare to go back to help ease the transition, according to Cancer and Careers.

Most people out on medical leave have had some contact with the office—at least with the people they get along with best . . . and the people who've been calling them frantically looking for the most recent version of Form XYZ. Start with these colleagues. Make sure you're up on the latest changes (and gossip). Play around on the computer to brush up your Excel or PowerPoint skills (or other techno toys). Consider attending industry events to keep your knowledge up-to-date while you're on leave. That way you won't walk into the office unaware of the latest trend that everyone is talking about and trying to handle.

You might also consider taking a workshop or seminar to update your skills. That's probably a particularly good idea these days, with today's ever-changing technology. It takes constant education to avoid becoming a Luddite. I say this as someone who is pulling herself kicking

---

5. "Healthcare Wide Hazards," U.S. *Department of Labor*, accessed December 4, 2013, https://www.osha.gov/SLTC/etools/hospital/hazards/ergo/ergo.html.

and screaming into the twenty-first century. Fortunately, I gave birth to my own little tech advisors, but not everyone plans so well.

Once you're ready to return, try to figure out a schedule that works for you, then discuss it with your supervisor. Hopefully you can come to an agreement that will keep everybody satisfied. Before you show up on the first day, you might take a look at your workstation to make sure it meets your current needs. Are you going to need more back support or a lower keyboard? If you have trouble reaching up, can you ask someone to rearrange the files so that the ones you use most often are in the lower cabinets? Don't forget ergonomics. Simple things like this can help you return more smoothly to the office environment.

And when you show up, focus on the work itself. Catch up on those phone calls and emails. Tackle the mountain of mail. Resuming your old routine can send the message that you're not just visiting to chat or check out your desk. You have made the transition from patient on leave to employee on the job. That will be reassuring for the others in the office and, in the end, will make it easier for you to put on your coat and head out the door at five o'clock.

What if you just don't want to stay? Then, maybe, it's time to look for a new job.

Frequently Asked Questions

Q: I don't want to sit home all day after I finish with treatment; I want to go back to work. Is that unusual?

A: Many, many people go back to work after cancer treatment. Some of them want to keep busy, some want to "give back," and some of them just need that paycheck. If you've taken medical leave, a company is required to give you back your old job. For more information on your legal rights, see Chapter 10: Legal Issues.

Q: Will people in my office be excited to see me return, or will they be looking for me to slip up?

Yes. And yes. People come in all different personality styles, and they react in all different ways to various activities. Some people are very supportive in general, while others are always on the lookout for something that might mean extra work for them. Unfortunately, you have to be ready for a whole spectrum of responses.

Q: Do I have to tell everybody in the office what happened? What about clients; do I have to tell all of them?

A: You are not required to tell anybody anything—except for whatever is involved in requesting time off or reasonable accommodations (see Chapter 10: Legal Issues). Some people are an open book, telling everyone all the details of their cancer treatment; others are completely closed-mouthed about it all, only sharing that it was a medical leave and that they're ready to be back at work. Many people, though, are in between. They tell some people (clients and colleagues) all the details, others get only a vague outline, and still others receive little or no information. It's a very individual situation. You have to think about what makes you feel comfortable.

Chapter 8

Looking for a New Job

Elissa Bantug, diagnosed with breast cancer at age twenty-three, was stunned when she finished treatment and was, essentially, dismissed by her doctor with a simple, "See you in a few months." She needed more information—and she was sure she wasn't the only survivor who did.

"I really wanted to get involved in making sure that cancer patients and survivors were cared for holistically," she says. Rather than sit back and hope things worked out better for others than they did for her, Elissa took action. She became involved with several boards as part of the Susan G. Komen Foundation and the Livestrong Foundation, as well as at her local hospital. "I wasn't one of those people who just sits on the couch."

Even all her committee work wasn't enough for the public health professional. "I wrote a grant with a medical oncologist at Hopkins to start the survivorship program at Hopkins." When the grant came in, Elissa made her move. She left her research position at the National Institutes of Health (NIH) for a new job: running the

Breast Cancer Survivorship Program at the Johns Hopkins Sidney Kimmel Comprehensive Cancer Center.

No longer a one-woman operation, Hopkins' Breast Cancer Survivorship program is now a multidisciplinary team of internists, oncologists, nurses, survivors, scientists, social workers, administrators, and researchers. The program helps survivors from the moment of diagnosis on and provides assistance with everything from pain management and fatigue to legal and financial issues and from sexual health and fertility to group and one-on-one counseling.

Elissa loves the new path she's on. "It's more than a job for me. It's not nine to five, Monday to Friday," she explains. "I like seeing people be able to get strength from one of the biggest adversities in their life," she says. "I see people at their worst and somehow get to their best in a very short period of time."

I know how Elissa feels. When I woke up from the all-consuming fog that is cancer treatment, I started to think about what I wanted to do with my second chance. Somehow the days seemed more precious, and I wanted to squeeze every ounce of joy and fulfillment I could out of every minute—while still devoting a considerable quantity of those moments to lying comatose in bed, recuperating. We talk about gratitude all the time, but, honestly, I had never truly understood the concept before. I turned my sights to writing more about health-care issues in an effort to make a difference in my own little way. (This book is part of that effort.)

I thought this was my own quirk until I read a blog entry by Margot Larson, lung cancer survivor and human resources consultant: "A traumatic life event may cause you to take an inventory of your life and re-align your priorities."[1] She probably thought she was talking about herself and her many clients over the years. But she was also talking about me. And about Elissa.

---

1. Margot Larson, "Changing Careers," *Journey of Hope* (blog), January 5, 2010 (3:40 p.m.), http://margotlarson.wordpress.com/2010/01/05/changing-careers/.

Redefining Yourself and Rethinking Priorities

Elissa was lucky, in a way. Her new purpose knocked on the door and announced itself to her. Not everyone, though, is so lucky. Most people have to systematically think about their lives to figure out what they want to do next.

To find out more about how survivors explore new arenas, I contacted Margot Larson, who had impressed me with her blog entry. She told me the story of a client who had stage-four lung cancer, which doesn't exactly carry a hopeful prognosis, and was working hard at a job she didn't like. The job wasn't interesting or enjoyable, and the workload was so demanding that she could feel it sap every last bit of energy from her. But the position came with a $20,000 life insurance policy that she wanted to be able to pass along to her children. While the client's instincts were maternal and commendable, Larson was concerned.

"I felt she was totally out of balance. She needed to really sit down and think," says Larson. "Wouldn't her children rather have her at home and a little bit stronger for a little bit more time than have the money?" Larson helped the woman think her situation through and realize that she was deciding which gift to give her children—the gift of money or the gift of herself, money or mom—and that maybe her decision needed a little bit more thought.

Sometimes it is hard to be objective about your own life, Larson points out. She recommends talking with a friend, a chaplain, a social worker, or a life coach. "You might need someone to think through your life priorities. You need to reassess and reinvent yourself." Friends can be especially helpful, Larson points out, because they usually know you very well; but you have to be willing to listen to what they have to say. And to do so, says Larson, "You have to go back to basics and really start thinking about what you want in your life and what is important to you."

Don't underestimate the power of a more objective voice, someone outside your own brain. "I can coach others; I feel good about

145

coaching others," says Larson. But when it came time to reassess her own priorities, Larson hired her own coach. "It's much harder to see the reality for yourself," she says. "But when I work with a coach, all she does is raise a couple of questions for me, and I've got it."

Larson recognizes that "we have to reassess where we are and what we want in our life—and what we don't want in our life." When Larson received her own diagnosis of lung cancer, she entered semi-retirement, and as of this writing, she is in a phase-one clinical trial. "My priority had shifted," she says. "My priority became taking care of my body, taking a good look at my lifestyle, and readjusting my life. I think it's very important to reduce the stress in your life."

That's why Larson switched from full-time consulting in human resources to part-time career coaching. "I was doing it all virtually, so I could do it on my schedule. I had my headset and clients I had never met." This gave her great control over the time in her life. "If I knew my treatments were the first week in the month, I'd wait until the second week in the month, and I'd pick a certain day and time that I knew would work for me," says Larson. That's when she set her appointments. "I continued to work because I needed the stimulation," says Larson. "I could use the money—that's for sure—but what I really needed was the stimulation." She was able to get that stimulus on a schedule that worked for the rest of her life.

Larson realizes, though, that making these decisions isn't easy for everyone. "I'm the sort of personality that is generally in balance." Making these adjustments is more of a challenge for many of us.

Here are some of the arenas that people think through:

Personal Values. Larson recommends making a list of your values and then ranking them in order of importance. These can include issues such as salary, benefits, commuting, work-life balance, service to others, flexibility, stability, prestige, and fun. None of these are all-or-nothing propositions. In my own life, for instance, I value the freedom of freelance work, but keep a part-time job so I that know I have at least some money coming in regularly. (Now if only I could find a part-time gig that pays a little more. . . .)

Strengths. Think about your strengths and weaknesses, suggests Larson. What do you enjoy, and what sorts of things do you hope never to do again? In my own life, I never even think about any job or freelance gig that asks about typing speed; I actually type something like eighty words a minute but—ssshhh—I don't ever want a job where my typing speed is valued more than my writing and editing ability; I want to spend more time exercising my brain than my fingers. (This preference goes back to the personal value of "fun.")

If you have trouble pinpointing your strengths, Larson suggests taking a look at any performance evaluations from work. You can also ask your supervisors, colleagues, and friends. Try to reflect on your skills and experiences more broadly than just your current or most recent position: think communication skills, not ability to summarize a meeting in clear bullet points; think analytic skills, not ability to pick the most appropriate furnishings for the office; think design, not laying out the company newsletter.

Larson recommends focusing on these broad skill areas:

- Creative problem solving
- Communication skills
- Persuasive skills
- Project management skills
- Creating rapport and building strong working relationships
- Motivating others and fostering a team spirit
- Technical and mechanical abilities
- Research skills

Think positively about your strengths; don't focus on deficiencies. "When I used to teach classes in doing job searches, people would say to me, 'I have no talent, I have no skills, nobody wants me,'" says

Larson. Now, positive thinking probably won't singlehandedly land you a job, but negative thinking certainly won't help. Talk to people who know you well—and then listen to what they have to say. They may well see qualities in you that you haven't noticed, or haven't seen as relevant.

For instance, when Larson was working in human resources, she did a little career counseling pro bono. Between her natural ability to talk with people and her expertise on the other side of the interview table, she was pretty good at it. One day, someone said to her, "Margot, why don't you get paid for this?"

She thought about it and decided that it was a good idea; she enjoyed helping people think about their careers, and, clearly, she was good at it or people wouldn't keep coming to her. So she decided to get some training and certification in outplacement services. "That way, I had all the proper training, the knowledge, on both sides of the table." These days, career coaching is most of what Larson does, all thanks to the friend who pointed out her skill.

Prioritizing. Larson recommends creating a chart that lists the top four or five priorities for your next job. For each item, note your requirements: the Reality (what you reasonably expect), the Minimum Acceptable (what you absolutely must have to avoid shooting yourself), and the Dream (the professional equivalent of winning the lottery).

For instance, Larson explains, you can easily figure out your financial minimum. Just consider how much you need to meet your mortgage payments, supermarket and power bills, and other expenses. Similarly, if you think about geography, you may decide you're willing to drive about fifteen minutes each way to work. The ideal would be a job located five minutes away, but you'd be willing to travel up to fifty miles a day—or maybe even one hundred miles; it's up to you. Plug that figure into your chart. You can also think about benefits such as health insurance; flexibility about when and where you work, including thinking about telecommuting one or two days a week; paid vacation and sick time; and so on. Looking at your chart, there are probably a number of jobs you can rule out from the get-go.

When you think about how happy you are in a job, says Larson, there are three basic considerations:

- The company you work for
- The job you do day to day
- The supervisor you have

It is helpful to distinguish between the three. Managers come and go, so as much as you may love your boss, it's important to be comfortable with the job and company as well. "We have a tendency to run away from where we've been," says Larson. People who have had a bad work experience may think they hate their job or their company, when really the problem is the boss. "You have to be careful about not letting the pendulum swing too far in the other direction when you're running away from something," cautions Larson.

"I worked with one woman who hated her job in a medical practice. So she said she never wanted to work in a medical practice again," says Larson. But when the woman thought about what she didn't like about the job, she realized that what really annoyed her was that she had no benefits and that nothing in the office was automated, so she was drowning in papers and files. What bugged her had more to do with the particular office than the overall environment of medical practices. This process helped her figure out where she wanted to work: in a twenty-first-century medical practice with reasonable employee benefits.

Once you figure out what is meaningful to you, says Tracy Fitzpatrick, Connecticut-based life coach and cancer survivor, you need to translate that into very practical actions. "For some people, it means finding new work. For some people, it means renegotiating what they have at work. For some, it means a new attitude about the work that they have." If you know what you're looking for, it's much easier to find it.

Building up the Nerve

For Rochelle, a survivor of a rare soft tissue cancer in her cervix, superstition held her back from looking for a new position.

"I stuck with a job that was literally making me ill," she remembers. She'd been working in an after-school program for more than two decades and had enjoyed it for quite some time. But recent changes in the parent board had created a toxic environment, especially because much of her job involved working with the board members. "The board made my life miserable," she says.

"I felt like damaged goods with the cancer, and how could I start something new when I had this thing hanging over my head?" says Rochelle. "I have always felt that scar on me." She felt as though she wasn't as strong or as capable as she had been before the cancer diagnosis and treatment.

Rochelle suspects that the board members knew that, too. "They could be as nasty as they wanted to because I wasn't going anywhere." They knew she would just plug along.

Not only did she feel like damaged goods because of the cancer; Rochelle was scared of change in general. Change had always been difficult for her, but cancer made that worse. "I feel like cancer puts you a little bit separate from the world. It's harder to be like everybody else. I feel like other people, people who haven't had cancer, are more carefree." Being a naturally nervous person, Rochelle felt that looking for a new job was tempting the fates, acting overly confident, almost like asking for trouble.

Eventually, Rochelle got up the nerve to look for another position. "It was just my time to move on," says Rochelle. "It was probably my time to move on a few years before I did. I stayed for seven years after I finished treatment. But I would say the last three years were increasingly difficult."

Here's the good news: Rochelle has since gotten a new job, with pleasant colleagues, a lovely work environment, and a location that is just a few blocks from her home. The moral of the story is that it's important to be gentle with yourself after cancer treatment. If you need some time before you're ready to look for a new job, take it. With a lot of work—and a little luck—it will all work out well in the end.

Sometimes the easiest first step, though, is to see if there are opportunities right in your own backyard.

Think about Your Current Office

"You're bored; that's normal. You're plateaued; that's normal," says Jansen, the career coach. "That's normal for everyone in their career," at some point, she says. There are probably lots of people who hated their jobs or their companies or their supervisors before they had cancer. Sometimes it's just taking the time to think about your job that makes you notice what had been true for quite a while.

So, maybe it's time to look around for something new.

Maybe you can start right where you are, suggests Jansen. Look around for other opportunities where you work now, before you explore outside the office. "Try to make your marriage work before going to find a new husband," she says.

If you've been working in an office, the people there already know you, at least a little bit. It's not just the folks you interact with every day. Other people have noticed you. You may serve as liaison with another department; you may have asked questions of someone outside your domain—or answered some. You may have sat in a company-wide meeting with people outside your department. Or you might just run into someone in the break room and compliment her new earrings. All of these people consider you familiar, at least to some degree. Certainly you're more familiar than someone who just walked in wearing a suit and carrying a briefcase.

When people look at a résumé of someone whose face they know, they're a little bit more comfortable than they are with someone who is just black ink on white paper. Assuming, of course, that you aren't known as the Person to Avoid in the office.

For starters, it's just plain easier to look around your current place of employment. You can do a little research without taking time off, and you can get a realistic feel for the position just by seeing whether and how often people doing that type of work have anxious looks on their faces. Plus, you have the advantage of knowing the corporate culture and how to operate within it.

"It's harder to look for a job in a new office," says Jansen. "What happens to people who've had cancer is that their confidence is not where it might have once been. They don't feel like they're at the top of their game." It's never easy to go on an interview; it's always nerve-wracking. But when you're feeling not quite yourself, it's even harder. So, consider the known environment first.

Jansen tells the story of a man she worked with at ESPN. He had been working in accounting and finance, and he wanted to move to a different department. Luckily for him, ESPN had a rotation program at that time, where employees could test out several other departments. It turned out that the man Jansen was working with really liked one of the spots he tried out, talent management, and was good at it. After the rotation program was over, he made a strong case for himself and was hired—you guessed it—in talent management.

"You never know," says Jansen. "I would never discount the possibility that you could move into another area. But you really have to build your case," she explains. It's easier in an organization where you are a proven entity.

Putting It All on Paper

When you are ready to start job hunting, you need that most basic tool: the résumé. As everyone knows, the résumé is your own personal sales brochure, minus the glossy pictures. It notes the jobs you've had, lists the accomplishments you've fostered, and highlights the education and skills you've acquired and honed. It's not all-inclusive; I've long since removed any reference to my high school job as ice cream scooper, as I'm really hoping not to be considered for a position that requires such expertise.

I'm sure you know the basics of putting together a résumé. But what you might not know is how to work around a gap in your résumé. You know, that time you may have taken off to recuperate from surgery, survive chemotherapy, schedule in radiation, or maybe just recuperate from the poison you'd been ingesting to fight cancer.

If you've stayed at the same company throughout treatment, you're golden whether you took time off or not. You were an employee for the entire time, so there's no reason to mention your medical leave on your résumé.

"You were there the whole year," says Jansen. "You don't need to create more problems for yourself by admitting that you went out on a leave. Then you'd have to start talking about why you went out on leave." Of course, that's everyone's biggest fear: that possible employers find out you were sick.

Consulting counts, too. If you did even a little bit of freelance work while you were in treatment, put it on your résumé. There's no need to mention the health-related impetus for your foray into self-employment. Nor do you need to point out that you worked ten hours per week instead of your usual forty-plus. Don't lie if you're asked, but there's no reason to bring it up unnecessarily.

If you're looking for a full-time job, you can always explain that you tried consulting but want to go back to regular full-time work. Employers might be relieved to know you got the freelance bug out of your system and are really looking to stick with a nine-to-five.

Even if there's still a gap in your résumé, there's no need to advertise your medical history. Consider using a different style of résumé: emphasizing the job title and skills rather than dates. More and more people are doing it, even without having the "C" word in their history. With this approach, you can simply list the years, not months, of employment. That way a gap of a few months is barely visible, or not visible at all. For instance, write:

Bookkeeper; Big Money Maker, Inc. 2010
Bookkeeper; Smaller Firm, Inc. 2011

Along the same lines, if you did some part-time work to keep yourself afloat during treatment, just list the job and dates. No need to mention whether you put in fifteen hours a week or forty. The point is to demonstrate the skills and work experience you offer. You can also highlight volunteer and community work; these efforts often involve plenty of skills, including multi-tasking, planning and organizing, and recruiting and working with volunteers.

Another approach to résumé writing is becoming more and more popular. Simply organize your work experience topically or by skill. I've done this for years, as soon as I noticed that people who wanted someone to write newsletters didn't care if you could write books (in fact, they worried that I would be too wordy) and people seeking ghost writers didn't want anyone with a "distinctive writing voice" (such as you might demonstrate in a magazine article). The theory, at least, is that a skills-based résumé enables potential employers to hone in on what they're looking for.

One more option suggested by Cancer and Careers is to use a non-traditional organization for your resume. You might list all of your skills at the top of the résumé, with bullet points that summarize your experience with each. Then, below that, you can briefly list the companies you've worked for with titles and years of employment. This, notes the Cancer and Careers website, is called the chronological/functional format. It, too, emphasizes what you want potential employers to know—your skills, education, and experience—while downplaying those persnickety little chronology details.[2]

---

2. "Minding the Resume Gap," *Cancer and Careers*, accessed December 4, 2013, http://www.cancerandcareers.org/en/looking-for-work/resume-gap.

Putting It Online

I am, as my daughter constantly reminds me, "very twentieth century" when it comes to technology. My phone is smarter than I am, and I tend to go on Facebook about once a year, to thank people for their kind birthday wishes. Often, I'm a month or two late. But I've learned that ignoring social media is kind of like conveniently forgetting about that twenty-page term paper that's due at the end of the semester: the issue doesn't go away—and, over time, can become an even larger hurdle.

When you're going through cancer treatment, people want updates. When's your next chemo? How was the last radiation? What's the latest on your rash-nausea-toenails-hair? A friend of mine who went through treatment in the 1990s told me she set up a phone tree to share the information; she'd call one friend and one family member with the latest news, and they'd take care of the rest. These days, that's a Luddite approach.

Whether it's reading the latest update on Facebook or the most recent posting on a blog (either long-term or set up for this specific purpose, such as through caringbridge.org), most people these days share their news electronically, to make it easy for friends and family to keep up and, arguably more important, to make it easy to disseminate.

The advantage is that this approach makes the information highly accessible. You don't have to update each person individually; it's open to all. In other words, anyone who can type can find out, for instance, if it is normal for your "chemo curl" hair to come back straight.

The catch is that friends and family aren't the only ones able to do a Google search about you. It's becoming increasingly common. And that plays into job searching more often than you'd think. Potential employers don't rely just on résumés, cover letters, and references anymore.

Here come the statistics: nearly two in five companies (37 percent) use social networking sites to research job candidates, according to a 2012 survey by CareerBuilder.[3] Just a few years earlier, in 2009, a study of employers that conduct online background checks found that 45 percent said they used social media to screen job candidates. The study found that employers tend to gravitate toward Facebook (65 percent) and LinkedIn (63 percent) to research candidates; a mere 16 percent use Twitter.

More to the point, about one-third (34 percent) of employers reported that they found something on social media that caused them not to hire a potential candidate. The most flagrant red flags, according to the CareerBuilder survey, were provocative or inappropriate photos (49 percent), information about drinking or using drugs (45 percent), demonstration of poor communications skills (45 percent), badmouthing former employers (35 percent), evidence of racial, religious, gender, or other types of discriminatory remarks (28 percent), and indications that the potential employee lied about qualifications (21 percent). So, you should try to avoid making these obvious mistakes.

Some "mistakes," though, are less obvious. That picture of your radiation rash or military hairdo that you posted on Facebook, or even the photo of your friends supporting you in the chemotherapy suite, might come back to haunt you. Not to mention your Life with Cancer blog or Twitter update on the results of your last blood test. As they say, once something is out there on the Internet, it's out there. The information wasn't intended for future employers, but they can access it.

So, what do you do? Some people's first response is to simply remove the possibly incriminating picture, posting, or email. That

---

3. "Thirty-Seven Percent of Companies Use Social Networks to Research Potential Job Candidates, According to New CareerBuilder Survey," *CareerBuilder*, April 18, 2012, www.careerbuilder.com/share/aboutus/pressreleasesdetail.aspx?id=pr69 1&sd=4%2F18%2F2012&ed=4%2F18%2F2099.

approach isn't infallible. If someone copied the post or picture and shared it with anyone else, it's still out there. I personally couldn't locate it, but people with a little more technological savvy can easily find that piece of potentially incriminatory evidence.

Other people decide to just ignore the whole virtual world, the theory being that if they don't post something about themselves, no one will. It's similar to the way toddlers assume that when they put their hands in front of their eyes, not only are you invisible to them; you can't see them, either.

"The knee-jerk reaction is often to run away and turn off and disengage from social media," says Joshua Waldman, social media strategist, speaker, and author of *Job Searching with Social Media For Dummies*. "Concepts like burying and hiding don't apply," says Waldman. "That's an old way of thinking about the Internet that's not relevant anymore."

"It's ironic, because the more that somebody disengages with their online reputation, the less control they have over it," he explains. "It doesn't go away because you close your eyes. It spirals out of control, and now, all of a sudden, you have no idea what that first impression's going to be."

The better strategy, says Waldman, is to post more and more. Drown out the bad with lots of good. Post articles you've written, do guest blogs, share some of your PowerPoint presentations with others. "Post more of what you *do* want people to know about you. Which, ideally, is not about surviving cancer but about the value that you're going to bring to your new organization," suggests Waldman.

What does that do to those medical updates? "It just pushes them down, pushes them down, pushes them down," says Waldman.

It's also very useful, says Waldman, to have a strong LinkedIn profile. LinkedIn.com is a business network designed to connect people with influential decision makers, potential customers, and colleagues. It functions kind of like a "virtual rolodex," if you remember what those are. "If you do your LinkedIn profile correctly, it's going to be the top page that comes up when someone Googles you," says Waldman. "And you're not going to put 'cancer survivor' on your LinkedIn profile."

LinkedIn can be useful, explains Waldman, but you don't have to jump on every social network bandwagon to get a job. You don't, for instance, have to start a Twitter account in order to get a job, he adds. Phew, thinks Beth the techno-newbie.

"The point is," says Waldman, "It's a net, so the more a person has out there, the greater the chances of getting caught." The stuff posted most recently is what comes up first on a search.

It helps to think about how recruiters use the online data, says Waldman. Some people recruit passively, which means that the recruiter or potential employer performs a search and a bunch of names—hopefully including yours—pops up. If this happens, we hope they'll see a nice online reputation, a good profile, some positive references, that sort of thing. It's a positive approach, but it's also passive and, therefore, hard to control.

More to the point, that sort of passive search is kind of unusual. Typically, people get referred by friends or family—folks who, almost by definition, know you've had cancer. "It's going to be hard to bury that online," says Waldman.

"I think that the focus is not necessarily to run away from that reality, but to simply overshadow it by the passion, [the] drive that's bringing somebody back to work," Waldman notes. You want to have that be the subject associated with your name on Facebook, Twitter, and other social media.

That process, says Waldman, is called pivoting. You can't really delete or change what's on the Web, but you can redirect your online persona, says Waldman. If you focus on the future and the value you can add to your next employer, that's what will pop up. And that, for cancer survivors, may well be the way to go.

But don't spend so much time with your online persona that it starts to replace your real-world networking. Landing the perfect job requires a combination of both.

Face to Face

Networking, résumés, and your online reputation may get you in the door, but then you have to make a good impression, to back up the sales pitch.

"People say, 'I'm finished with treatment; I have not worked in two years. How do I explain that? Do I discuss it in the interview?'" Larsen explains. "The answer is: NO."

An interviewer does not have the right, legally or otherwise, to ask medical questions in a job interview. He or she can only ask whether you are capable of performing the essential tasks of the position. And you are required to answer honestly. But the Americans with Disabilities Act (ADA) specifically prohibits employers from asking about any disability. Cancer qualifies. (For more information on your legal rights as a cancer survivor, see Chapter 10: Legal Issues.)

It is probably best, suggests Cancer and Careers, to speak in general terms about your experience and focus on the future, rather than the past.[4] If a question comes up, say, about a gap on your résumé, it is useful to have a simple sentence that you've practiced. You don't want to be caught off guard.

Some options are as follows: "I was dealing with some family issues, but they're all resolved now." Or, "I was consulting for a while, but realized I am happier in a corporate environment." Or even, "I was unhappy with my position and took some time to figure out what I wanted to do, and I've realized that Your Company, Inc., is a great fit for me."

That future-oriented comment is key. The goal is to turn the potential employer's attention toward the contributions you will be able to make in the next day, week, or year. You can think about

---

4. "Job Hunting After Cancer Treatment," *Cancer and Careers*, accessed December 4, 2013, http://www.cancerandcareers.org/en/looking-for-work/Job-Hunting-After-Cancer-Treatment.

saying something like, "At this company, I will be able to apply my analytic skills to contribute to your important research."

When you have your response ready, consider doing a mock interview with a friend or a coach. You can practice your "gap explanation" and your "future-oriented" comments. If you can say them to a friend without giggling, chances are you'll feel confident in an interview.

Illegal Questions

Illegal or not, every so often, some people will ask inappropriate questions. The key is not to lie, but not to provide "too much" information. Larsen recommends answering those questions graciously and with humor, but without offering information. "For instance, if someone says, 'I see your hair is very short—have you been sick?' you might respond, 'I'm perfectly healthy today. And I can give you the name of my hairdresser if you'd like.'"

Plenty has been written about the importance of dressing the part when you go on an interview. "It addresses image," says Margot. For people who've been through cancer, though, that means rethinking their interview wardrobe, even if you've been doing this for a while. Just because something looked good on you before you were diagnosed doesn't mean it's going to work now.

Many people gain or lose weight in cancer treatment. Make sure your clothing isn't too tight or too loose. Try not to display scars, if you can help it. And if your breasts aren't symmetrical, find a jacket (or something else) that will disguise it. You don't want to give anyone a reason to wonder whether you've been ill.

Another topic to consider, suggests Larsen, is that people often look kind of pale when they are going through and recuperating from treatment. In my case, people kept giving me make-up— lipstick and blush and things I couldn't identify. I don't normally wear make-up, so I wasn't sure what was going on; was this meant as an insult or a helpful bit of advice? Because I didn't know what to do with the stuff, I ended up donating it to a battered women's shelter. But most people aren't as clueless as me—and make-up, I am told, can hide a multitude of "sins," including, apparently, a cancer experience.

Another way to look less wan, the approach I take, is to wear a splash of bright color, particularly by your face, to lighten up a grayish countenance. Remember, you want to look your best as you are now, says Larsen. It's all about looking to the future, not the past—the future with a new and exciting career opportunity.

Frequently Asked Questions

Q: How do I decide if I want to go back to my old job?

A: This can be a complicated decision; sometimes it is helpful to talk it through with a friend, colleague, therapist, or coach. Think about how your needs and interests have changed as a result of going through cancer diagnosis and treatment—and whether you think your familiar work environment will suit the "new you."

Q: When I'm looking for a new job, do I have to put "cancer treatment" on my résumé? What if there's a gap in my employment?

A: Human resources experts and career coaches recommend not mentioning the "C" word. It can spook employers and potential employers who often take one look at the word and see employee absences and rising health insurance rates in their future.

Q: What about in an interview; should I mention that I had cancer?

A: Again, experts recommend keeping mum on the subject. Of course, the choice is yours. But it might be easier to either avoid displaying a gap on your résumé altogether or explain it with a well-practiced, forward-looking phrase. Perhaps, "I was dealing with some family health issues, but that's all in the past now. I am looking forward to . . ."

Q: What do I do if there's stuff online about my cancer history? Will possible employers see it?

A: It's pretty hard to completely hide something that's already on the Internet. You can try to delete or change it, but usually if it's out there, someone who's determined to find it probably can. The best thing to do is to add lots of career-focused material "on top" of the cancer-related posts or tweets. Try to make sure the first thing that comes up when someone Googles you is exactly what you want them to see: a great article you wrote, presentation you organized, or recommendation you received.

Chapter 9

Switching Careers

Ann Ogden lived a high-excitement, high-pay life as a fashion designer. She was born in the UK, and her work took her all across Europe and Asia. She spent twelve years in Paris, in addition to frequent jaunts to Italy as well as to Japan, China, and Korea, checking out factories and fabrics and such. She enjoyed her travels, grabbing time to experience the various cultures and, especially, her love of food. Eventually, she ended up in New York, bringing her British accent along with her.

In a sense, the fashion industry was a bit of a mismatch. Ann came from a long line of chefs and master bakers. "My family has always been in and around food, and I traveled a lot as a child with my parents. . . . I've always had a very broad taste in food," she explains. Though being comfortable with trying new places, foods, and other things did prepare her in some ways for the life of a fashion designer: "I loved to eat and cook, and it was a really great experience to live and work in these kinds of places," she says.

Ann didn't let her 2001 diagnosis of kidney cancer slow her down. Luckily, the only treatment necessary was surgery, and as soon as she was back on her feet, she was back in the office—and on the road. "A lot of my job was about travel," she says.

Then, four years later, she was diagnosed with breast cancer, a second primary. Triple negative.

This time, she was subjected to what she calls "the slash and burn of cancer treatment." A lumpectomy followed by chemotherapy, followed by radiation treatment. Because she developed an allergy to one of the chemo drugs, the treatment itself lasted for almost a full year. "I got my diagnosis in February and had my last radiation on Christmas Eve." The best holiday gift you can't wrap.

Because Ann couldn't travel during treatment, she took a break from work. "I did a few small jobs, but basically decided to go through treatment without working. I was lucky to be able to do that," she says, acknowledging that not everyone has that opportunity. "I gave myself up to my treatment."

Eating was a challenge for Ann, as it is for everyone going through chemotherapy. But her culinary knowledge and willingness to experiment saved her. "When my taste buds became all crazy, I was able to adapt the food that I was eating. I would tweak things, and I could focus on the things that tasted good and forget the other stuff."

Ann talked about her approaches in her support group, sharing stories and trading recipes. The more she talked with other cancer patients, the more she learned how fortunate she was to know so much about food.

"A lot of people had gotten used to eating in restaurants," she says. "It was incredibly hard for them to find things that they wanted to eat because their favorite chicken noodle soup from the diner tasted disgusting." Their comfort foods weren't soothing, nothing tasted quite right, and they didn't know how to adapt the food. When you're going through cancer treatment, the last thing you want to do is tackle a major new subject like gastronomy.

Ann found that a lot of people didn't know much about food. "I think for women of my generation, there's a kind of strange disconnect from the kitchen," she says. "There is no joy in cooking."

And, too, empty nesters often feel as though there's no need to bother; why cook for one or two when you can simply forage in the cabinets or order in? "But then you get out of the habit and everything becomes difficult," Ann noticed.

She found she really enjoyed sharing her secrets, recipes, and cooking tips with the people in her support group. She wanted to share her knowledge, starting with the things that got her through treatment, such as apple blossoms in water to make that vital liquid more palatable and the poached chicken recipe that her friends called "miracle chicken."

These informal conversations evolved into little cooking classes, where Ann taught what she called "some really 101 things." For example? "How to make kale taste good, for instance. How to prepare cabbage, how to cut a carrot, how to sauté things—when the onions are ready, that sort of thing," says Ann.

Teaching about food was a fun and productive way to spend her time in cancer treatment, Ann thought. But as she reached the end of treatment, she started to think about what she wanted to tackle next.

"I wasn't sure what I wanted to do," she remembers. "Having spent time away from my fashion career, I didn't really want to go back to that. I wanted to do something with people," she recalls.

Having time off to think really helped her focus on what she wanted, in a way that even the initial jolt of her kidney cancer did not. "I had two second chances," says Ann. "I ignored the first one." But she wasn't going to ignore the second.

She decided she really enjoyed teaching cooking and wanted to make a full-time gig of it by starting her own not-for-profit organization. But having only worked in the corporate world, she didn't really know how to do it. She typically worked *for* someone— she wasn't used to running the show.

She started by writing a business plan. "I showed it to a friend of mine who's a retired businessman," Ann says. "He said, 'This is great.'" Ann was relieved; at least she was starting off in the right direction.

Then the friend did something totally unexpected—he gave her the seed money to start the nonprofit. "I wasn't expecting that. I just wanted him to look at the plan and make sure I was going in the right direction."

Now, about eight years later, despite a recession-based bump in the road, Ann's organization, Cook For Your Life!, has really taken off. It develops and teaches nutrition and cooking classes for cancer patients, survivors, and caregivers. Ann focuses on helping her students eat more fruit and vegetables and use healthier cooking techniques.

The classes are great, too. As a culinary novice, I've taken a few of Ann's classes. Each time, a small group of us—patients, survivors, and caregivers—worked together on a variety of dishes. I learned that I'd been cutting vegetables all wrong, and got a lesson in proper knife work. I also garnered a few new recipes and some education in foods that are helpful in fighting cancer.

Plus, as we cooked, and then ate at a long, wooden table, I got to spend a few hours with a group of people who all understood the cancer experience. I was impressed that a fashion designer had found a way to combine culinary education and cancer support into a yummy afternoon.

Cook For Your Life's website is pretty impressive, too (www.cookforyourlife.org/). It allows people to search for recipes not only by the foods in their refrigerators, but also by what stage they are in the cancer process or how they're feeling that day. "If you need a bland diet, you can find recipes for that; if you're fatigued, you can find a whole bunch of very simple things to do," says Ann. They also have specific categories of recipes for chemo, radiation, nausea, and healthy survivorship.

But Ann still wasn't satisfied with just these activities. "In my classes, I used to get a lot of middle-class white ladies coming and not much else," Ann remembers. "I wanted to help people who were really left out of the equation."

Ann decided to focus on Latino cancer survivors. In New York City, that meant developing courses geared toward Puerto Ricans and Dominicans, for whom there was little material available. "There was a lot of stuff that was culturally appropriate in California, but that's Mexican-oriented, which means nothing to the Dominicans or Puerto Ricans or Ecuadorians who live here," explains Ann.

After she'd been offering these classes for a few years, Ann was approached by a researcher at Columbia University's Mailman School of Public Health, who was interested in doing research with Hispanic breast cancer survivors and food. The researcher wanted to find someone who was already working with that population and, ironically, the white British lady was the only person she could find.

"It was mind-blowing to me, too," Ann laughs. Together they applied for—and received—a National Institutes of Health (NIH) grant. And they've been researching and offering classes ever since.

Cancer totally changed Ann's life. "I went from fashion designer to helping people learn to cook kale to working with Columbia University on an NIH-funded project," Ann notes, proudly. "From a high-paying job to a much lower-paying one. But I am so much happier." Ann is sticking with Cook for Your Life! for the long haul; as she says, "fight cancer with your fork."

Khit made her change a little earlier in the career-building process. She was still in undergraduate, taking pre-med courses. "I have a brain, I love school, I love helping people," she explains. "I always knew I wanted to be a doctor."

But then she went to talk with her academic advisor. "My advisor said, 'I really don't think you should take your MCATs. You should go into nonprofits.'"

"You're crazy," Khit responded.

"Khit, that's all you do," the advisor pointed out. "If you get into medical school, you'd have to quit Imerman Angels for three years."

THE CANCER SURVIVOR HANDBOOK

Bear in mind that Khit works upwards of eighty hours per week for Imerman Angels, a nonprofit organization that pairs people touched by cancer with a survivor of the same type of cancer.

"I couldn't do that," she said to her advisor.

"When I thought about that, it made me have so much anxiety; I realized there's no way that I can *not* do what I do," says Khit. "That was my aha moment."

Khit made a change. "In February of this year, I changed my focus from applying to med school to a nonprofit bachelors degree." When she finishes, Khit may not get a job at Imerman Angels, but she knows what type of work she wants to do. "I just love teaching people how to be involved in an organization, whether it's Imerman Angels or something for diabetes or abused women," Khit says.

Some people, though, make a shorter-term career change as a result of their cancer experience.

Short-Term Career Change

When Sherry was diagnosed with ovarian and endometrial cancer, she'd been struck by how little women—herself included—knew about ovarian cancer and its risks. She thought that someone should really do something about that, about public education on ovarian cancer. At the time, she was a high-level manager in a Washington, DC–based nonprofit organization devoted to Native American issues. A member of the Oglala Lakota Nation, Sherry had worked for several Native American organizations, ranging from health-care to financial issues, and also had served on a number of boards of directors. Unlike Ann, though, she knew her way around the world of nonprofits.

As she went through treatment, Sherry joined a support group of cancer patients. Through this group, she attended an Ovarian Cancer National Alliance (OCNA) conference and started to receive their newsletter. A few years after she finished treatment, Sherry read in the newsletter that they were looking for an executive director.

"I thought that would be a great opportunity for me to try to spread the word about the prevalence of and risk factors for ovarian cancer. So I interviewed for the job, was selected, and made a commitment to the board to stay three to five years," she remembers.

Given Sherry's management experience and expertise and her interest in the area, it was a perfect fit. "I was passionate about getting information out to women and seeing what I could do to educate people," she says. Under Sherry's watch, OCNA saw the passage of Joanna's Law, the Gynecologic Education and Awareness Act, which promotes public knowledge about ovarian cancer, its risk factors, and its symptoms. "You can't get a law through without having a great grassroots network," Sherry notes.

The organization also increased its network of volunteers and expanded its program of teaching medical students about the cancer experience. By the time Sherry left, the program reached physicians assistants and nurse practitioners as well. And she got the organization on a somewhat stronger financial footing. After about three years at the ovarian cancer organization, Sherry found that she missed working in Native American issues and resigned from OCNA to return to work for a Native American organization.

Not everyone, though, has a new career call out to them, as it did for Ann and Sherry. Most people have to figure out what they want that new career to be.

Finding the "New You"

"Sometimes when you're emerging from that process—whether you have a chronic illness or are finished with treatment—you don't necessarily want to go back to the life you were leading before," says Tracy Fitzpatrick, life coach and cancer survivor. You may realize that your priorities or interests have changed, she suggests. Or you may notice that you haven't been happy at work in a while, and the jolt of a diagnosis encourages you to rethink your choices. Cancer and treatment takes away your sense of control, so, sometimes, when that's all done, people want to grasp more control over their lives.

The first step to making a change, of course, is figuring out what sort of change you're looking to make.

Right after you've finished treatment can be a good time to rethink your life, says Tracy. "It can be a really good timeframe for asking those questions about meaning and integrating some of the experiences of cancer and doing some design about what you want in life now," she explains.

"I've seen a lot of people make very radical changes in their lives, and I've also seen people go back to a very similar life but with a new attitude," says Tracy. "And they've gotten a lot more fulfillment out of their lives because of the internal shift, not because they've changed circumstances."

Tracy recommends that people start by taking their emotional temperature and tune into their sense of energy, engagement, and curiosity. She asks her clients to keep track of when they feel most excited and engaged with life. That wouldn't be when, for instance, they just read the same paragraph several times and still don't know what it was about or when they had a brief conversation with a neighbor but tuned out for the entire ten minutes.

As we saw in Chapter 1: Now What?, it can help to think about what makes you feel "alive." Feeling "alive" can happen at major events such as a college graduation, the birth of a child, or a marriage proposal. Or it can be much smaller moments, such as strolling through the park and noticing a blue jay, laughing hard at a silly joke, or playing peek-a-boo with your friend's toddler.

Now, Tracy doesn't mean that these "alive" moments are just happy ones. "You can have a real sense of engagement and a good cry at the same time," she explains. It can happen when you're reading a book or watching a movie that moves you to tears or talking with a friend about a job loss or diagnosis that really moves you, makes you feel truly engaged with life.

The next step, says Tracy, is to stick that experience, those experiences, under an emotional microscope. "Think about what particularly engaged you about that conversation," says Tracy. "Was it that person, and how did you feel about that? Or was it the environment you were in? And what was the content of the experience—was that what engaged you?"

Occasionally, this approach leads to unexpected revelations. "Sometimes someone will come to me for the first session and say, 'Oh my God, I'm so miserable in my job, I can't stand it,'" says Tracy. Then they monitor their feelings day to day, and it turns out that they really enjoy about two-thirds of their job. It's just the part where they're dealing with so-and-so or doing a particular task or sitting in a half-day meeting that's the problem—a big enough problem to make them want to throw out the proverbial baby with the bath water. "This approach can help people get very astute about the situations they're in now and about themselves," Tracy adds.

Sherry, for instance, found that after she finished treatment, she really wanted to devote some time to working on cancer awareness. She enjoyed the day-to-day activities of nonprofit management, but she wanted to bring her skills to bear on the Ovarian Cancer National Alliance.

It also helps to think about the accomplishments that you find most meaningful. For me, I found that completing a master's thesis and getting my advisor's stamp of approval is much more significant than receiving a piece of parchment while wearing a cap and gown. I feel good about researching and writing and about accomplishing a goal.

A good friend of mine centers her life around her relationships; she'll look back at a good day as one where she had a few meaningful interactions with friends or family, whether or not she checks anything off her to-do list. Another friend is highly competitive; a good day for him is when his sales statistics are higher than those of the others on his team (even if they all did better the previous week).

You can also look for a way that your work can add meaning to your life. The catch is to figure out what "meaning" signifies to you. Here are some ways that people often find meaning in their work, according to Cancer and Careers (CEW). Do you want work that

- Offers new opportunities
- Provides the chance to gain knowledge, understanding, or expertise
- Imparts financial reward
- Offers recognition
- Provides the opportunity to express or live by certain values or principles
- Offers access to an exciting or intriguing industry or field
- Provides the opportunity to change or improve something
- Provides an academic or analytic challenge to solve problems or answer complex questions
- Allows a change or modification in lifestyle, priorities, or relationships
- Provides opportunities to innovate or create
- Allows you to contribute to a cause or a social or political movement[1]

If you think about what sort of "meaning" you are looking for, it might help you figure out what you're interested in.

A friend, relative, or life coach can be very helpful in this process. They understand the issues involved in figuring out a new career and can be an objective observer, asking provocative questions from what Tracy calls an "observational platform." As Fitzpatrick explains it, "A coach does not give advice about how to live life. A good coach, I think, helps guide someone through a process that helps them connect with their own passions and their own value system

---

1. "Finding Meaningful Work," *Cancer and Careers*, accessed December 4, 2013, http://www.cancerandcareers.org/en/looking-for-work/finding-meaningful-work.

and what has meaning for them and become an astute observer and decision maker in their own lives." It can help people learn about their own wishes and yearnings and passions.

Some people find it useful to go through this process in a group setting. "It works great when people are doing it in a group together and are talking about it. They talk about each other's experiences," says Tracy. That interaction can lead people to new insights about their own lives. The goal is to achieve a level of wisdom, self-knowledge, and confidence.

There is one caveat with this approach, though, Tracy notes. It does not work for someone who is clinically depressed. "But if someone is mildly kind of down, this actually works really well at helping them connect with themselves," she says.

Learning to Network

Informational interviews are nothing new. But people usually think of them as a way to find a new job, not a new career. They can also be helpful when you're rethinking your career path.

Tracy typically recommends that survivors have between five and ten open-ended conversations with people as they explore. Ask people what they do on a daily basis, what they like best, and what they put off until the last possible minute.

When you finish the conversations, take a few minutes to assess your response. Were you excited by what you heard; can you picture yourself doing those functions day after day? What parts of what you heard made you want to join in, and what made you want to crawl in a hole and disappear? "Follow that sense of engagement and that sense of, 'Wow, I would hang out here in my spare time, forget being paid,'" says Tracy. "If you follow that feeling, you're going to find good work." Work that you find meaningful and enjoyable.

Ann tested out her new career just by working with friends in her support group. She wanted to work with food and with cancer survivors. The catch is that she figured out exactly where she wanted to work, but it didn't exist yet.

Once you determine where you want to go, you have to figure out how to get there. "And sometimes it takes many steps and years to make that change," says Tracy. "Other times, oftentimes with people in midcareer, it's not that difficult because they've amassed a bunch of skills and experience that they have to repackage, but they still have a lot going for them to make a change into a new field. It may be that at age fifty, it's hard to become an astronaut at that point," she says. "But many changes are possible."

That's not to say that it's an easy process for anyone, especially in a challenging economy. It can be very frustrating. "Most adults don't like to be learners," says Tracy. "A one-year-old will fall a thousand times while he or she learns to walk. But that's not how we adults like to learn." But entering a new area requires a period of being the new kid on the block—not always a comfortable spot.

Then there are the rejections. True, you only need one job—but sometimes you have to get rejected and reject a lot of gigs to get to that one. I like to remind myself that F. Scott Fitzgerald, C. S. Lewis, Madeleine L'Engle, Agatha Christie, and even Dr. Seuss and J. K. Rowling were rejected by publishers before they eventually went on to change the literary landscape. (Now, if only I could sell half as many books as any of them.)

Tracy suggests remembering that you're not a beginner at life—you're just doing something brave to try to enter a new arena. And you bring strong skills, education, and experience—not to mention plenty of enthusiasm.

Avoiding the Gremlins

Tracy points out that the path to someplace new is littered with gremlins. Everyone has her own specially designed gremlins.

"Sometimes your gremlin will get you to edit a piece a billion times before you show it to anyone," Tracy explains. While there could well be a grain of helpfulness in there, sometimes it's just overkill. I know my elephant-memory gremlins force me to create my own deadlines in advance of my editors' deadlines, to give me an extra day or two for fretting over commas.

What to do about those gremlins? Well, it's easier said than done. Tracy recommends that you don't listen to the beasties and just trust yourself. The first step is to recognize who's worrying about the job, you or the gremlins.

Those gremlins have another technique, notes Tracy. They can keep you distracted by fomenting little battles.

- "I should have done this" and "No, it's all right."
- "I should have kept my mouth shut" and "It's a good thing I said something."
- "That typo will ruin my career; no one will ever hire me again" and "My editor fixed it, told me I'd made her day, and went on with her life."

Back and forth, back and forth. Frustrating, time-consuming, and not particularly productive.

I try to remember what Tracy says: don't waste your precious time and energy on those gremlins. Even when you're combating a dangerous combination of chemobrain and venturing into a new environment. Cultivate your inner ally, the cute little imp who says, "OK, so what can you learn from this? And, isn't it time to move on?"

That imp? She's my new best buddy.

Changing careers, especially when you've devoted years to one profession, can be a scary prospect. But once you've faced down cancer, and what's a little job hunt? The key is to figure out what you want to do, and where you want to do it, and then formulate a plan to get there. Break the massive undertaking down into little steps and get rid of the gremlins, and it's much more manageable—not to mention rewarding.

Frequently Asked Questions

Q: Is it usual to consider switching careers after cancer?

A: Often, cancer is a jolt that forces people to rethink their lives, including their jobs.

Q: How do I figure out what I really want now?

A: Focus on what experiences make you feel most "alive," either positive or negative. Then analyze what about those experiences really matters to you. Sometimes talking with a friend, therapist, or coach can help.

Q: What do I do about those little voices that keep reminding me of everything I've ever done wrong?

A: Send those gremlins to bed. Try to spend more time with the little imp who helps you figure out what you can learn from those mistakes, instead.

Q: I am midcareer—is it possible for me to start a new career?

A: Midcareer people have developed a large range of skills and expertise. It's a matter of packaging that experience in a way that applies to the new direction you seek.

Chapter 10

Legal Issues

Barbra had just finished legal training when she joined a Florida law firm as a litigation paralegal. The firm was small, and each lawyer had an assistant. She was assigned to a lawyer who had somewhat of a reputation within the firm.

"He'd been through fifteen paralegals in the past two years," Barbra says a colleague warned her in her first few days on the job. But Barbra seemed able to weather the bumps and work it out. Besides, she liked her other colleagues and most of her clients.

Then—after five years of working in that position and receiving several raises—she found a lump in her left breast. And she was diagnosed with breast cancer.

Though Barbra had been living in Florida for many years by this point, she decided she'd rather be treated at Dana Farber Cancer Institute, a National Cancer Institute (NCI) hospital up in Boston. She spoke with the lawyer she worked for, and he told her to "do what you have to do."

So Barbra made arrangements to head north and had the IT department set up a computer. "I figured I'd be going back and forth for about three or four months," she says. She could draft documents and pleadings and submit them through the Internet. Every so often, she would go back to Florida to go to court with clients.

But Barbra was sicker from chemotherapy than she'd anticipated, there were unexpected complications, and she ended up being able to work fewer hours than she'd hoped. "There were about two weeks where I couldn't even log onto the computer and do any kind of work," Barbra says. She tried to stay in touch with her boss by telephone and email, but he wasn't good about responding to her updates and questions.

Then one day, she got a FedEx package saying that she was terminated. Her boss didn't come right out and say that Barbra was fired because she had breast cancer, of course. That would be blatantly illegal, and, after all, it *was* a law firm. Instead, the lawyer talked about how his clients were suffering because his paralegal wasn't as available as usual.

Barbra was stunned. "It was really devastating," says Barbra, "because here I am, fighting to save my life, and here's this guy who says, you're out of here."

Barbra focused on her treatment and getting better. She eventually hired a lawyer and was granted a small settlement from the law firm. "I felt like my boss really messed up my life," she says. Now that she's healthy again, she needs to go back to work. It would be much easier, she says, if she could return to her old job in a familiar environment, with responsibilities and procedures she knows well and colleagues who are also friends. Unfortunately, that's not an option. So she's looking elsewhere.

Chris has a similar story, though with a happier ending.

He was a thirty-three-year-old cyclist when he was diagnosed with testicular cancer. He was serving in the military—and he had to fight to keep his job. "Anybody who gets cancer in the military gets a medical review board. But I think most people don't realize the significance of that."

"Basically, three military doctors review your medical records and, depending on what they decide, you could be medically retired," explains Chris. Most civilian jobs don't force you to retire after you have been through a life-threatening illness. Fortunately, the review worked out fine, and Chris kept his job.

But a few years after Chris finished with treatment, he was promoted to a special operations unit as a flight test engineer. "Flying aircraft was part of the gig," he explains. To get clearance, he saw the flight surgeon, had all his records checked. All routine.

"Then I got my records back with a big red X on it that said 'not clear for flying.' And that was a problem since my job was to fly an airplane," Chris remembers. Apparently the issue was outdated medical information. "The doctor in charge of the decision was an older doctor, not up on all the current literature," says Chris. "He had an old book with older treatments for testicular cancer," he says. And in that book, the chemotherapy was much harsher, and the prospects of lung cancer and other similarly worrisome long-term effects was much greater. "Treatment had come a long, long way since that medical book was written," says Chris.

Chris lodged a formal protest with the military. "Thank God, I had relationships with some of the top doctors in the world." He got his physicians to write letters testifying that Chris was fine and that there was no cause for concern. "I had my lungs tested and all that kind of stuff," he adds. Then Chris submitted his new records and crossed his fingers.

"My records came back, and the big red X had been taken off of it, and it said 'cleared for flight,'" Chris recalls. "The doctor was actually insulted that I had questioned him—and that I was right." Chris took the special ops job and stuck with the military until he retired—on his own terms, and with full benefits.

It's hard to believe that even in the twenty-first century, people can still lose their jobs because of cancer. Fortunately, there are a few federal laws in place—supplemented by a variety of state laws—that help protect jobs while people are in treatment, and after.

The Rules

Legal issues can become very complicated, and the details are key. While there are some federal laws, such as the Americans with Disabilities Act (ADA) and the Family Medical Leave Act (FMLA), there are also state equivalents, which vary across the country. As Joanna Morales, Esq., CEO of Triage Cancer, explains, it is vital to investigate the laws around your situation.

"My first recommendation to people when they're looking into these issues is to do their research," says Morales. Much as you study your medical condition and delve into the treatment options and their risks, you should also look into how all of this—the cancer, the treatment, and the recuperation process—will affect your ability to work and to hold down a job (which, as Chris and Barbra demonstrate, are not always the same thing).

You may find that the issues are fairly complicated. If so, you may need to consult a lawyer or a legal organization about your particular situation (see Appendix 1: Resources for Survivorship for more information). Please note that this chapter is no substitute for professional legal advice.

Anticipating the issues is important. Experts suggest that you start by thinking about how cancer and its treatment will affect your work life. Can you schedule your treatment around work? Will you be incapacitated by chemotherapy and need to take that time off? Do you anticipate a need for flexible time to fit in radiation treatment and check-ups? Will you experience extreme fatigue, skin or temperature sensitivity, or other side effects that might make it hard to work the way you have been? What have people who've gone through this line of treatment done in terms of their work? How quickly will the symptoms dissipate and when will you reach your "new normal"?

Next, you need to find out about your options and benefits at your job. Some companies, typically larger ones, have a human resources department and documents that outline company policies, benefits, insurance, time-off policies, and other details.

Most legal questions that arise for survivors in the workplace come in one (or more) of five types:

- Disclosure
- Time off from work
- Reasonable accommodations
- Discrimination
- Health insurance

There is occasionally overlap across these issues and the laws that address them.

Disclosure

Deciding whether to tell people about your cancer diagnosis is very personal. Some people share the news with everyone they run into, while others keep their mouths zipped tight, even among people they work closely with. Donna, for instance, told her supervisor, colleagues, and students about her diagnosis and treatment; Lisa's colleagues, on the other hand, never had any idea that anything unusual was going on.

Often, though, people fall somewhere in between.

When you think about it, sharing cancer news isn't any different than telling people about any other personal information. You wouldn't run up and down the halls telling everyone about a broken printer; you would probably only mention it to people whose job functions require using or repairing that particular electronic device. You wouldn't blab the story about your lousy blind date to everyone you come in contact with; that's the sort of story you save for your good friends. Those are probably the types of relationships you consider—professional and personal—when you think about sharing the cancer diagnosis.

In addition to thinking about your personal communication style, you also need to consider the professional environment you work in.

If, as Morales says, you know your employer has a horrible history of discrimination and treats people with serious conditions very poorly, you might not want to say anything. On the other hand, if your employer is a cancer survivor or the relative of one, and has a fantastic track record of supporting employees through difficult times, then maybe you would be comfortable talking about your situation.

"If you have decided that you want, or need, to share your diagnosis, you should approach your employer in a way that feels comfortable to you," says Rebecca Nellis, vice president for programs and strategy at Cancer and Careers, a nonprofit organization that advises people on managing their disease and jobs. The key is to think it through, not just react on the spur of the moment. Consider your own communication style, your work relationships, and the office environment—and what will work best for your situation.

No matter how tight-lipped you are and no matter how awkward the work situation, you will need to tell someone if you plan to request time off or reasonable accommodations to your work schedule or conditions. As you think about how to do this, focus on what you want to disclose, when you want to disclose it, how you want to tell people, and who you want to tell. All these decisions are very personal. What worked for your best friend over in accounting may or may not do the trick for you.

"I would definitely recommend thinking through the conversation beforehand and deciding what information, and how much information, about your diagnosis you are comfortable sharing," Nellis adds.

What to Disclose

Generally, you don't have to share information about your medical situation with an employer or potential employer unless you choose to. Certain circumstances, though, might encourage you to choose to share that information. Specifically, if you are asking for some type of medical leave or reasonable accommodation at the job, you'll have to show why you're entitled to it. Employers don't take any more kindly to "because I want to" than do parents of petulant toddlers.

But sharing information about your medical condition to show that what you're asking for is legitimate doesn't entail a blow-by-blow description of chemo-induced vomiting, tingling fingers and toes, or radiation burns. In fact, says Morales, you don't even necessarily have to say (or write) the word "cancer."

"The laws differ in terms of what you have to share and the way you have to share it," says Morales. "But, generally, you don't have to provide a diagnosis if you are concerned about disclosure."

For instance, under the Family Medical Leave Act (FMLA), which focuses mostly on ensuring time off from work without job loss, the U.S. Department of Labor provides model certification forms that many employers use.[1] The form requires a health-care professional to provide certification of the medical need, and that professional must list his or her practice or specialty area along with contact information. The model form provides a list of health-care professionals who are qualified to provide the certification.

Before you ask a health-care provider to fill out the form, think about how much you are willing to share. "If you ask your oncologist to provide the information, you're kind of giving away the diagnosis," says Morales. If you ask your internist or family practice doc, on the other hand, you're not sharing as much information.

When to Disclose

People can—and do—raise questions about disclosure at any time: during the job interview and application process or while you're already working at the job. In general, though, you don't have to disclose more than you want.

---

1. http://www.dol.gov/whd/forms/WH-380-E.pdf.

Thanks to the Americans with Disabilities Act (ADA), a federal civil rights law passed in 1990 designed to protect people with disabilities from employment discrimination, a potential employer can't ask about a disability or require an applicant to take a medical exam before making a job offer. ADA covers companies and agencies with more than fifteen employees and applies to employees who have an impairment that substantially limits one or more major life activities. In case you were wondering, cancer qualifies as an impairment.

Potential employers, according to the Equal Employment Opportunity Commission (EEOC), can't ask an applicant any of these questions:

- Will you need a reasonable accommodation to do this job?
- Have you had cancer?
- Do you have a disability that would interfere with your ability to perform the job?
- How many days were you sick last year?
- What prescription drugs are you currently taking?[2]

Of course, that doesn't necessarily simplify things. If you are asked one of those questions in an interview, you have to do some quick calculating. Is this a teachable moment? Should you explain that the question is not relevant to your qualifications for the job and the employer shouldn't be asking it under ADA? If you do that, there's a good chance you won't get the job, and, as Morales points out, you might never be told why.

At the same time, you should also think about whether you would be comfortable working for someone who is either unaware of basic employment law, or simply lacks compassion—or whether you are just OK with answering the question.

Either way, it helps to think this out in advance. You should know your attitude ahead of time and plan out your approach in advance

---

2. "Enforcement Guidance," *Equal Employment Opportunity Commission*, July 26, 2000, http://www.eeoc.gov/policy/docs/guidance-inquiries.html.

of the job interview. Come up with a sentence or two to answer any questions and practice saying them out loud a few times so that you can say them comfortably. That way, whatever you do, it will be a considered decision, not a knee-jerk reaction that you may come to regret.

What if an interviewer asks about a gap in your résumé? "You could answer in the following ways," suggests Nellis:

- "I was dealing with a family issue that is resolved now, *and* I am thrilled to discuss how my management skills can build the team and grow your business."
- "I realized that what I was doing didn't fulfill me, so I took a step back to think about what would make me happy, *and* I think my tech background would really be an asset, not just for this role but for the company as a whole."

Whatever you choose, be sure to emphasize that all the issues are resolved and you are now ready and eager to get back to work— preferably at the job under discussion.

It is important, notes the U.S. Department of Labor, to always be truthful about your medical situation, though, as we've said earlier, that doesn't mean overly forthcoming. Some people feel that they're being dishonest if they don't explain everything about their disability.

But it is your choice—you are not legally required to disclose your diagnosis. If you do, all you need to share is basic information about your condition, limitations, and any accommodations you might need.

If an employer does know that an applicant has a disability—perhaps because it is obvious or perhaps because the person has voluntarily mentioned it—it is OK to ask if that disability might pose difficulties in performing a particular job task, says Morales. Then, if the applicant says that an accommodation might be necessary, the employer is allowed to ask what accommodation would be needed. The employer can, obviously, consider this information in his or her decision.

Once you've received a job offer, an employer may ask questions about your health (including any disability) and may ask for or require a medical examination—but only if *all* applicants are treated the same way. In other words, employers can make these requests only if *all* employees are asked the same questions or are required to take the same exam.

That's equally true if you are dealing with an employer that you're already working for. In that case, though, be careful to get out in front of any difficulties and disclose in advance of any issue. It's better to disclose your disability and request accommodation before your job performance suffers or problems occur. If an employer issues a disciplinary notice or action, then finds out about the disability, the employer doesn't need to rescind that action, says EEOC. Employers also don't have to lower their performance standards for someone with a disability. That's why you ask for reasonable accommodations, so that you can continue to perform the essential functions of the job. So it's important to disclose as soon as you realize that you are having difficulties on the job, *before* it becomes a problem for the company.

By the way, an employer can't blow your cover. If you don't want your coworkers to know what's going on, cancer-wise, your boss can't share the information—even if people ask why you're getting what they might see as "special treatment." According to EEOC, if an employer tells co-workers that someone is receiving a reasonable accommodation, that amounts to a disclosure of the employee's disability and goes against the letter (as well as the spirit) of ADA.[3] Instead, the employer should focus on maintaining employee privacy—and, possibly, do some organization-wide training on the requirements of EEO laws, including ADA.

How to Disclose It

Fortunately, the rules about how to disclose aren't that complicated. Your request doesn't have to be formal. You don't even have to

---

3. "Questions & Answers about Cancer in the Workplace and the Americans with Disabilities Act (ADA)," *Equal Employment Opportunity Commission*, accessed December 4, 2013, http://www.eeoc.gov/laws/types/cancer.cfm.

make the request in writing, according to EEOC. Nor do you need to mention ADA or even the term "reasonable accommodation."

Now, an employer *is* allowed to ask for "reasonable documentation" about the disability, according to EEOC. Employers are entitled to know that the person has a disability that is covered under ADA and that the requested reasonable accommodation is, well, reasonable. If you ask for more than one accommodation for the same disability, that's fine; some people require only one reasonable accommodation, while others may need more than one. But the employer is allowed to ask about each request.

"It is very important in any conversation at work to be true to who you are and to explain that your treatment is a fluid process and that this is what you know today but that it could change," says Nellis. "And then be prepared to keep the people who need to be updated updated," she adds.

Who to Tell

Deciding who you want to disclose the information to is another issue you should probably think out in advance.

First, check out company policy. Many employers have their own in-house procedures that detail how to handle accommodation requests. The employee handbook or your company intranet might have this information.

If the company has a human resources (HR) department or an Equal Opportunity Office (EOO), that office might be able to help. Many people, though, just speak directly with their manager or supervisor.

In general, the U.S. Department of Labor states that people with a disability such as cancer are entitled to be able to:

- Feel assured that the information about your diagnosis and treatment is being treated confidentially and respectfully
- Learn about the hiring practices at any organization
- Choose to disclose your disability at any time during the employment process—or not at all

- Receive any reasonable accommodations needed for an interview
- Know that employment decisions are based on your skill and merit

By the same token, people with a disability are responsible for

- Disclosing the need for any work-related reasonable accommodations proactively, before any problems occur
- Sharing skills and experience on the job
- Being truthful about the diagnosis and treatment
- Being upfront about any difficulties you are experiencing on the job and thinking creatively about any reasonable accommodations that would help[4]

In general, reasonable accommodations aren't set in stone. As Morales explains, "Reasonable accommodations are things that are specific to that individual and the medical conditions that they have and the person's particular job responsibilities."

Time Off from Work

The Family Medical Leave Act (FMLA) of 1993 is the only federal law that allows people to take time off from work while protecting their jobs. So, typically, when cancer survivors need time to go through or recuperate from treatment, they turn to FMLA, though sometimes time off can be considered a "reasonable accommodation" under ADA.

Basically, FMLA guarantees that eligible employees can take up to twelve weeks of unpaid leave. You can use this leave all at once or in bits and pieces, even as brief as a few hours at a time. It also guarantees that employees will maintain their health insurance while out on leave; if the company had been paying the premium, it is still responsible for payment. Arguably the best part of FMLA is that employees

---

4. "Youth, Disclosure, and the Workplace Why, When, What, and How," *U.S. Department of Labor*, accessed December 4, 2013, http://www.dol.gov/odep/pubs/fact/ydw.htm.

are guaranteed to be able to return to the previous position or an equivalent job with the same salary, benefits, and other conditions of employment, according to the U.S. Department of Labor.

Eligible employees are those who have worked at the organization, be it a private company, government agency, or school, for at least twelve months (at least 1,250 hours) over the most recent twelve months.[5] FMLA doesn't apply to all companies, only to those that have fifty or more employees within a seventy-five mile radius. Unfortunately, these days, that rules out a number of businesses.

Often, though, states offer ADA equivalents that extend these benefits to smaller employers. The easiest way to find out about these laws is through the state Department of Labor. It is entirely possible that you might qualify for FMLA under both state and federal law. But, as Morales explains, "You can't stack the state twelve weeks on top of the federal twelve weeks."

When you ask for time off, you don't have to mention FMLA specifically, according to the Disability Rights Legal Center. Your employer can ask you to get medical certification from your doctor or another health-care provider, though you have fifteen days to do so. Your employer can also ask for all sorts of information—the name, address, telephone number, and fax number of your health-care provider; the provider's area of practice/specialization; and information on symptoms, diagnosis, hospitalizations, doctor visits, prescribed medications, referrals, and other ongoing treatment.[6]

Usually, this is a note, often on letterhead, that is signed and dated by a physician and states

- That you have a serious illness
- When the illness started

---

5. "FMLA Frequently Asked Questions," *U.S. Department of Labor*, accessed December 4, 2013, http://www.dol.gov/whd/fmla/fmla-faqs.htm#3.

6. "Medical Certification for the FMLA and ADA," *Disability Rights Legal Center*, last modified September, 2011, http://disabilityrightslegalcenter.org/sites/www.disabilityrightslegalcenter.org/files/Medical%20Certification%202011.pdf.

- Whether you will need time off continuously or in short blocks of time
- Whether you will need further treatment after the absence

Remember, you only have to disclose enough information to support your need for medical leave. Also, as we've seen, your oncologist does not need to be the one to provide the medical certification. You can ask another member of your health-care team to do so if you want to keep the diagnosis private.

You may need to supply an update on your medical certification or a second opinion in order to keep your FMLA rights. But, according to the Disability Rights Legal Center, the employer is required to pay for that second opinion. And if the first and second opinions differ, you'll need a third opinion, which your employer must also pay for.

As with everything else, you may need to consult a lawyer about your particular situation.

Reasonable Accommodations

As we've said before, a person can ask for a reasonable accommodation for a disability such as cancer at any point—during a job interview, at the job offer, or after five years on the job. That doesn't mean that an employer has to grant every request, nor even that an employer must provide the specific accommodation requested.

An employer can claim that a particular accommodation will result in undue hardship, which means that it creates too much difficulty or expense for the particular company. The most appropriate accommodation is probably one that employee and employer agree on. ADA doesn't require any particular method of deciding on an approach to reasonable accommodation, so some companies have developed their own protocol.

The U.S. Department of Labor's Job Accommodation Network (JAN) website offers a six-step interactive process that brings employer and employee to the table to figure out how to deal with a person's disability in a way that works for everyone involved.[7] JAN, which is part of the Labor Department's Office of Disability Employment Policy, is actually a really good resource for anyone dealing with the after-effects of cancer, as it offers free one-on-one counseling as well as numerous documents. The six steps are as follows:

Step 1: Recognize an Accommodation Request. We've already talked about the process of disclosing the medical condition. Once an employee tells the employer what is going on, the employer should make sure the request is clear, act quickly to prevent a problem from occurring, and assign someone to be responsible to make sure the accommodation is achieved. Often, employers conduct some sort of HR training for managers and supervisors so that they know how to work with a person who discloses a disability.

Step 2: Gather Information. The next step is for the employer to learn more about the situation. JAN recommends that employers ask the employee for information; the person with the disability is probably best suited to help figure out the limitation and what accommodation or accommodations will work best. Employers should be careful about asking for medical records and only request what is absolutely necessary. The JAN website offers this warning: "Asking for all medical records will rarely, if ever, meet this test."

Step 3: Explore Accommodation Options. This is where employer and employee brainstorm—and it's often helpful when you, the survivor, walk in with specific suggestions. Chances are you know more about your limitations, and your strengths, than anyone else. It helps for everyone to keep an open mind throughout this process.

---

7. "JAN: For Individuals," *U.S. Department of Labor*, accessed December 4, 2013, http://askjan.org/indiv/index.htm#on.

8. Beth Loy, "Accommodation and Compliance Series: Employees with Cancer," *U.S. Department of Labor*, last modified March 4, 2013, http://askjan.org/media/Cancer.html.

The JAN website (www.askjan.org) makes some specific suggestions, based on the type of disability and limitation.[8]

Fatigue/Weakness
- Reduce or eliminate physical exertion and workplace stress
- Schedule periodic rest breaks away from the workstation
- Allow a flexible work schedule and flexible use of leave time
- Allow work from home
- Implement ergonomic workstation design
- Provide a scooter or other mobility aid if walking cannot be reduced
- Provide parking close to the work site
- Make sure materials and equipment are within reach range
- Move workstation close to other work areas, office equipment, and break rooms
- Reduce noise with sound absorbent baffles/partitions, headsets, etc.
- Provide alternate work space to reduce visual and auditory distractions

Medical Treatment Allowances
- Provide flexible schedules and/or flexible leave
- Allow a self-paced workload with flexible hours
- Allow employee to work from home and/or provide part-time work schedules

Respiratory Difficulties
- Provide adjustable ventilation and avoid temperature extremes
- Keep work environment free from dust, smoke, odor, and fumes
- Implement a "fragrance-free" workplace policy and a "smoke-free" building policy
- Use fan/air conditioner or heater at the workstation

Skin Irritations
- Avoid infectious agents and chemicals
- Avoid invasive procedures
- Provide protective clothing

Stress

- Develop strategies to deal with work problems before they arise
- Provide sensitivity training to coworkers
- Allow telephone calls during work hours to doctors and others for support
- Provide information on counseling and employee assistance programs

Temperature Sensitivity

- Modify work site temperature or provide an office with separate temperature control
- Modify dress code and use fan/air conditioner or heater at the workstation
- Allow work from home during extremely hot or cold weather
- Redirect air conditioning and heating vents

Step 4: Choose an Accommodation. If the interactive process produces more than one possible accommodation, you might have to pick. It's nice when the employer selects the accommodation that you prefer, but he or she might just pick the easiest or least expensive approach. If you're not sure whether a particular approach will work, you and your employer can agree to test out the accommodation for a set period of time, and then revisit the discussion to make adjustments.

Some employers might want a written agreement about a "test accommodation," outlining the length of the trial period and what will happen if the accommodation doesn't work. That way, if and when the subject comes up again, no one is surprised.

Step 5: Implement the Accommodation. This might seem obvious, but it's certainly a step you don't want to skip. If the accommodation involves equipment, make sure the equipment is installed correctly and that you understand how to work it. If it involves a change in scheduling, everybody involved should be aware of the change.

If the accommodation requires an outside service involved, someone has to take responsibility to make those arrangements. If the accommodation involves a job reassignment, your employer should give you some time to adjust to the new situation. It's often helpful to have one person assigned to make sure the accommodation happens without a hitch.

Step 6: Monitor the Accommodation. It would be nice to think that once a change is made, everything else flows easily. Alas, life sometimes interferes with the best of intentions. Sometimes the employee's limitations change (e.g., you get stronger the further out you get from chemotherapy treatment), the workplace equipment changes, the job itself changes, the workplace itself changes (perhaps the company switches from closed offices to cubicles or moves to another location altogether), or the accommodation becomes an undue hardship for the employer.

As with any other workplace issue, communication is key: the employer should tell the employee if it becomes too difficult to maintain the accommodation, and the employee should tell the employer if a problem arises or, better yet, if the accommodation is no longer necessary.

For more information on the interactive process, check out www. askjan.org.

Discrimination

Cancer is a protected class, which means hiring and firing decisions cannot be based on that information. If they are, the person can bring a lawsuit against the employer.

That being said, proving discrimination is a tough one, says Morales. Usually, it is easiest to work these issues out informally. "In these situations, in an employment context, it's almost never useful to go to court," she explains, "unless you have a fantastic case. Like a case where your employer put in writing, 'We're firing you because you had cancer,'" says Morales. The chances of that happening are pretty slim; employers have become fairly savvy about what is, shall we say, kosher and what is not.

Remember—your medical information must be kept private and in a separate location from your personnel file, according to the Disability Rights Legal Center.

When it comes down to it, says Morales, there are legal options and then there are practical choices. "A lot of times, talking to people about their practical options is much more relevant to the conversation," says Morales. She asks, "If your employer is discriminating against you and making your life miserable at work, do you want to keep that job, or do you want to go somewhere else?"

Health Insurance

Health insurance has been a challenge for cancer patients and survivors in several ways. But, picture a law in a mask and cape: the Affordable Care Act (ACA) of 2014, which was signed into law in March 2010. While the health-care law doesn't offer free and unlimited coverage for everyone, it will make the situation much easier, especially for cancer patients and survivors.

The health-care law is being phased in bit by bit, and we should feel its full effects in 2014.

In the world before the Affordable Care Act, health insurance companies in many states could deny coverage to individuals who have pre-existing conditions or disabilities—such as, say, cancer. If insurance was available for someone with a pre-existing condition, the surcharge may well have been prohibitive; companies could charge what they liked to cancer survivors. Or the insurance company could search for an error, or some other technical mistake, on a customer's application and use this error to deny payment for services when you got sick.

As a result, coverage for people living with conditions such as cancer has often been priced out of the reach of most Americans who buy their own insurance. Unfortunately, many self-employed people just choose to let their insurance lapse altogether.

Even if you get insurance through your employer (or your spouse's employer), you may find that an insurance company can exclude coverage for a pre-existing condition for a period of time—sometimes as long as twelve months. Again, it depends on the state. A year is a long time for a cancer patient or a survivor to wait for treatment or follow-up tests. The choices could be shelling out more money than you earn in a year or holding your breath for twelve months while you wait for your pre-existing condition to time out.

There were a handful of states, such as New York, that legislated that health insurance firms cannot turn down patients with expensive conditions such as cancer. Even so, those states have allowed the insurance companies to raise their rates on high-cost patients. In other words, even if insurance has been available to you, the cost may have pushed it out of reach.

People who did have access to health insurance and could afford the premium and co-payments may also have found that they were subject to a lifetime dollar cap. That cap, notes the U.S. Department of Health and Human Services, would have limited how much the insurance company would be willing to pay over the course of your entire life. Under this system you may be going along, receiving treatment and follow-up care, and—if you live long enough—find out that you have run out of health insurance coverage. Not ideal.

The federal law is intended to address many of these issues.

The way it stands now, the Affordable Care Act will guarantee health-care insurance for cancer patients and survivors; insurance companies will not be allowed to turn people down because they have a pre-existing condition or disability. They won't be able to kick people off the insurance plan when they become ill. Health insurance companies won't be able to raise rates because of a pre-existing condition or disability. In addition, the anticipated federal law will eliminate annual and lifetime caps for coverage. Some preventive services, such as mammograms, screenings for cervical cancer, and colonoscopies may even be free. Cross your fingers.

Under the Affordable Care Act, insurance companies won't be able to raise their rates on what feels like a whim. For the first time ever in every state, insurance companies will be required to publicly justify any rate increase of 10 percent or more. Those premiums must go to providing health care, not funding fancy marketing campaigns or executive perks. Insurance companies will have to spend at least eighty cents of your premium dollar on your health care or improvements to care. Or pay out a rebate to customers.

Another advantage of the act, at least in theory, is that people won't feel stuck in their jobs because of the need to maintain health insurance. If you start a new business, change jobs, move to another state, or retire early, you will still have access to affordable health insurance. There will be an Early Retiree Reinsurance Program (ERRP) so that employers can continue to provide benefits to retired workers who are not yet eligible for Medicare. So you will have the ability to think about what you want to do next—and do it without worrying about maintaining your health insurance.

The catch is that everyone will have to carry health insurance, or pay a fee. If affordable insurance isn't available, there may be funding or tax credits to help cover the cost.

The truth of the matter, though, is that it is hard to know exactly how the Affordable Care Act will, in the end, finally fall out. Be aware, though, that as of 2014, the options and functioning of health-care insurance will change, probably for the better—especially for cancer patients and survivors.

Frequently Asked Questions

Q: Should I tell people at work that I have cancer?

A: Every situation is individual. Think about your personal style, your relationships with colleagues and clients, and the work environment when you're trying to decide. The key is to make a conscious decision, based on what you think will work best for you.

Q: Do I have to tell my boss or a prospective employer that I have had cancer?

A: No, you are never required to tell anyone at work that you have had cancer, much less give information about your exact diagnosis, treatment, or prognosis. The catch is that if you need to request time off or reasonable accommodations on the job, you may have to reveal limited information—just enough to "prove" the need. But you don't ever have to say the "C" word if you don't want to!

Q: What are the laws involved that can protect me at work?

A: The major federal laws that can help cancer patients and survivors take time off and make reasonable accommodations are the Americans with Disabilities Act (ADA) and the Family Medical Leave Act (FMLA).

Q: I work at a small company with about thirty employees. Do these laws still help me?

A: The FMLA does not apply to companies with fewer than fifty employees. But some states have laws that do; check on the local situation.

Q: What does ADA address?

A: ADA protects workers with disabilities—including cancer—from workplace discrimination. It enables people to request "reasonable accommodations" from their employers.

Q: What does FMLA address?

A: FMLA helps people take time off from work, while maintaining their health insurance coverage, without jeopardizing their jobs.

Q: Is the Affordable Care Act going to mess up my insurance?

A: Hopefully not. The truth is that we don't know for sure how it will all play out. Cross your fingers.

Section 3

Wellness Issues

When I was diagnosed with cancer, I felt like I lost all control over my life. I couldn't trust my body anymore. If I wanted to feel safe again, if I wanted to be able to plan for weddings and graduations and other life events, I had to follow the advice of my cavalcade of oncologists, surgeons, radiologists, and other health-care providers. Every minute was scheduled, and when I wasn't sitting in some doctor's waiting room, I was taking care of my kids, doing laundry or food shopping, or trying to work. Or, better yet, grabbing a (not so quick) nap.

I felt like I no longer had jurisdiction over my own life.

I wanted to regain that sense of control. I wanted to do something to continue to fight cancer, but on my own terms. One way I found—and continue to find—I could regain my feeling of independence is to focus on wellness.

Lindsey, who was diagnosed with leukemia two days before her twenty-fifth birthday, feels the same way. She has found that using "alternative" modalities has given her a sense of control over her life—a sense that she had lost throughout her two and a half years of cancer treatment. "At a certain time, after all this treatment, when

I began seeing my doctors only about once a year, I decided it was time for me to take control of my own health," says Lindsey.

Exercise and nutrition, Eastern medicine, and complementary modalities can increase strength and energy, heal a myriad of side effects, and help prevent recurrence or the appearance of a new cancer. In general, all cancer survivors should rethink the way we eat and how much and often we exercise. After fighting off a deadly disease and, perhaps worse, surviving cancer treatment, our bodies aren't as energetic and strong as they were before we were diagnosed. Thinking carefully about what we feed them and how we strengthen them can do a lot to improve our quality of life. Other "complementary modalities," ranging from reflexology to journaling, can help, too.

Regaining a sense of power over your life is very important for psychological well-being. Shelley E. Taylor, professor of health psychology at UCLA, suggests that even the "illusion" of personal control can be beneficial. Specifically, she suggests, studies have shown a relationship between a sense of control and better psychological health as well as better physical health outcomes.

Dr. Stuart Vyse, the psychology professor from Connecticut College, has found similar results. "When you are a cancer patient, much of the treatment and what happens is done by other people," he says. "You show up to the appointments, but there's not a lot of emphasis on what you personally can do to help combat your disease."

When you finish treatment, it helps to have a sense of control. "I think that's why alternative therapies are so popular, especially among people with various medical conditions," says Vyse. "Because whether they work or not, they do supply a sense of control because they're something that you choose to do rather than something your doctor is telling you to do."

As holistic energy practitioner and teacher Annalise Evanson says, "Wellness is really about living a fulfilling life."

Chapter 11

Survivorship Care Plan

Elissa Bantug was a twenty-three-year old researcher at the National Institutes of Health (NIH), focusing on risk-taking behavior among adolescent girls, when she was diagnosed with breast cancer. Treatment was rough, no surprise. But Elissa *was* surprised by how thrown she was when treatment was over.

When she finished her last radiation treatment, Elissa talked with her medical oncologist, asking him what was next.

"Nothing," he said. "Have a nice life."

When she asked her internist, he said, "Well, what did your oncologist say?" When she followed up with more specific questions about diet and exercise, the doctor just looked at Elissa as if she were crazy.

But wait a minute, she thought. There were so many unanswered questions. "I wanted to know what to eat, how to exercise, what to do with the rest of my life, how to care for my emotional well-being," Elissa remembers. She wasn't ready to be out there on her own.

Like Elissa, many cancer patients get "lost in transition" between active care and post-treatment care. When we finish with surgery, chemotherapy, or radiation, there is no longer anyone thinking regularly about our health, our functioning, or our sense of security and well-being. We're on our own.

A New Philosophy

These days, there's another possibility. About a month or so after the final treatment, be it chemo or radiation or even surgery, your doctor calls you in for a little chat, explains Matthew J. Matasar, MD, MS, who is an attending physician in the Adult Survivorship Program at New York's Memorial Sloan-Kettering Cancer Center. Matasar is on the forefront of this new approach called a "survivorship care plan."

"The doctor might say, 'Congratulations, you're in remission. Treatment is behind you, and there's a good chance that you've been cured,'" says Matasar.

"Then the doctor would outline the strategy going forward, saying something along the lines of this: 'I'm going to do this surveillance for a couple of years, and if the disease hasn't come back by then, I'm going to back off even further, and then at five years, if we're having the same kind of conversation, chatting about your work and the kids and such, then at that point I'll be letting you go, releasing you into the wild,'" explains Matasar.

Matasar is not only a practicing oncologist; he also conducts research on survivorship and care plans. He feels that preparing a person to transition from being a patient to being a survivor is very important. "If someone goes from seeing a doctor regularly to being handed off to a primary care physician, that can elicit a little anxiety in the patient and a sense of betrayal or abandonment," he explains. "One patient told me that at the end of treatment, he felt like Wile E. Coyote," Matasar says. "He felt like he kept running and running, and then he looked up and suddenly there was no ground underneath him. He'd walked off a cliff like a minute ago and didn't even know it."

Instead, handing over the survivorship care plan can serve as a graduation ceremony of sorts. "Patients get the assurance, the comfort of knowing that they're done and that they're OK," says Matasar. There's no black cap or gown, alas. "I tell them that this is a virtual flipping of the tassel."

As with any graduation, of course, there's a sense of completion and of pride in that completion—and, at the same time, a little bit of uneasiness about the unknown that follows. But with a care plan, survivors at least have the medical equivalent of a map and compass.

Matthew, who had brain cancer in his early twenties, really wishes that survivorship care plans had been around when he was going through the process. "That would basically have meant that I would have had a Sherpa guide through my entire journey to help my parents and me navigate insurance and discuss what was unique to me."

Trying Not to Get Lost in Transition

How did this approach come about? The Institute of Medicine (IOM), together with the American Society of Clinical Oncology, produced a report called *From Cancer Patient to Cancer Survivor: Lost in Transition*, which pinpoints the problem. Perhaps more important, the report lays out a solution: the need for providing each cancer patient with an individualized survivorship care plan when she finishes treatment.

The plan should provide a full record of the care the patient received, as well as outline what the patient can expect in the future, both in terms of medical monitoring and long-term effects of the treatment. The President's Cancer Panel has jumped on the bandwagon and endorsed the idea of a survivorship care plan as well.

The other equally important part of the survivorship care plan, notes the Institute, looks toward the future. It identifies the person or office that will be coordinating all continuing care. It lays out the necessary follow-up care and any increased risk that survivors may face. For instance, female Hodgkins survivors who have chest radiation are more likely than the average woman to have breast cancer and need appropriate monitoring.

Survivorship plans should probably have three basic parts, according to the IOM. They should

- Describe the treatment received.
- Outline plans for future tests, scans, and examinations, including surveillance for recurrence, spreading, or future cancers.
- Address intervention for the myriad consequences of cancer, including medical problems such as lymphedema and sexual dysfunction; symptoms, including pain and fatigue; anxiety and depression among survivors and their caregivers; and concerns related to employment, insurance, and disability.[1]

These plans, notes the IOM, should also pass the baton cleanly. Survivors should know who is in charge of their medical life after cancer. In fact, the IOM recommends that health-care providers have a formal discussion of this plan with people as they move from patient to survivor.

Going Component by Component

Survivorship plans are serious documents, but they're not exactly doorstop material. "They don't need to be so overly detailed," says Matasar. In fact, the lymphoma survivorship care plan form used at Sloan Kettering is just a handful of pages. Length is not the most important thing, says Matasar. "The plans need to be 'individualizable.'"

The first part of the plan, which outlines your personal cancer history, should be detailed enough to provide any future health-care person with all the information you need. Wouldn't it be nice to not have to remember what surgery took place on which day? According to the IOM, the survivorship care plan should include

---

1. "Cancer Survivorship Care Planning," *Institute of Medicine*, November 2005, http://www.iom.edu/~/media/Files/Report%20Files/2005/From-Cancer-Patient-to-Cancer-Survivor-Lost-in-Transition/factsheetcareplanning.pdf.

- A list of all diagnostic tests performed and their results.
- A description of the tumor characteristics (noting sites, stage and grade, hormonal status, and marker information).
- Dates of when treatment started and was completed.
- A summary of all the treatments given, including surgery, chemotherapy, radiotherapy, transplant, hormonal therapy, gene, or other therapies provided. This section should list all agents used and provide the treatment regimen, total dosage, and the identifying number and title of clinical trials (if any). It should also note any indicators of treatment response and toxicities experienced during treatment.
- A description of all psychosocial, nutritional, and other supportive services that the patient received.
- A list of the institutions and health-care providers involved, with full contact information.[2]

Basically, the first component, the treatment summary, outlines "what I did to you," says Matasar.

A patient who has been taking assiduous notes throughout the process might well have all of this information. But how many cancer patients can actually do that?

I know I was overwhelmed. First, I'd been diagnosed with cancer, which, in and of itself, is enough to monopolize your brain cells for quite some time. Then there was the schedule which, when paired with my physical limitations, accounted for much of my day. I'd take the kids to school, go to the doctor's office—whichever one— and then rest up before I had to pick the kids up and take them home. Somewhere in there, I had to do laundry, manage to feed my children on a regular basis, and try to earn a living. And now I'm supposed to remember all of those details?

---

2. Ibid.

So far, I've been able to answer most of the medical questions that doctors have asked about my treatment. But there's no guarantee that I have everything at my fingertips when I need it.

The second component of the plan should prepare survivors for the plethora of appointments and tests lying in wait. According to the IOM, this section should outline:

- How the survivor is likely to recuperate from the toxicities of treatment, including any need for ongoing health maintenance or therapy.
- A list of the types of cancer screening and other tests and check-ups the survivor will need, including a schedule and notation of who should provide them.
- Details on the possible late and long-term effects of the cancer treatment and the symptoms of these effects.
- Information on possible signs of recurrence and second tumors so that the survivor can keep an eye out for them.[3]

My doctors are responsive, knowledgeable, and very professional. They have given me all this information—but verbally. So, when chemobrain (or should I call it "normal aging?") kicks in, I can't remember if the six-month appointments will continue for five years or ten. It would be nice to have a document to refer to.

The third part of the plan aims to help survivors with all those pesky "late effects" of cancer and its treatment. It should cover everything from the risks of another cancer or heart disease to how to cope with difficulties in bed to the importance of preventive care, such as quitting smoking and limiting alcohol consumption. It outlines when a survivor needs her first colonoscopy or breast MRI, plus any psychosocial needs. These issues include the following:

---

3. Ibid.

- Facts about the possible effects of cancer on marital/partner relationships, sexual functioning, work, and parenting. The report should also address the potential future need for psychosocial support.
- Information on the potential insurance, employment, and financial consequences of cancer and, as necessary, referral to counseling, legal aid, and financial assistance.
- Specific recommendations for healthy behaviors, such as nutrition, exercise, healthy weight, sunscreen use, virus protection, and preventing osteoporosis as well as the benefits of smoking cessation and cutting down on use of alcohol.
- When appropriate, the report should recommend that the survivor discuss with their immediate relatives about any increased risk and the need for cancer screening; for instance, having a mother or sister with breast cancer increases your risk of the disease.
- As appropriate, information about genetic counseling and testing to see whether the survivor could benefit from more comprehensive cancer surveillance, chemoprevention, or risk-reducing surgery.
- If suitable, the report should also include information about effective chemoprevention strategies, such as Tamoxifen for women at high risk of breast cancer or aspirin to help prevent colorectal cancer.

Possibly the best part of the plan is that it names a point person for any further questions.

Don't Forget about the Rest of You

It took me about two years after I finished with treatment for my Hodgkins disease before I got around to having a Pap smear. After all, I hadn't had any trouble with my woman parts. Besides, it meant making yet another appointment, hanging out in yet another waiting room, and seeing yet another doctor. While I could get up the energy to see my internist, ophthalmologist, and even dentist, somehow—for reasons that don't make sense even to me—I drew the line at seeing a gynecologist.

The truth of the matter is that I had my next Pap smear when, for insurance reasons, I had to find another internist and my new one did Pap smears. I know, I know; I write about health-care issues. I know the importance of regular screening. What is my problem? Fortunately, the test came back negative.

It turns out that I'm not the only cancer survivor with doctoritis. Many cancer survivors may be very diligent about going to all their follow-up appointments with their cancer docs, but not everyone is so good about returning to their internist for those basic flu shots, cholesterol screenings, bone density tests, and other "routine" matters.

Unfortunately, having had cancer doesn't give you a "get out of health care free" card. In fact, oddly enough cancer survivors should be just as concerned with their general health care, including any ongoing issues, as they are with cancer. So while we may feel very connected to our oncologists (and I know I do), we can't ignore those internists or family practice docs.

A lot of people become attached to their oncologists because they see these doctors as having saved their lives, says Claire Snyder, PhD, associate professor of medicine at the Johns Hopkins School of Medicine. Survivors become so attached to their onco docs, says the researcher, that they may not reconnect with their primary care doctor.

"Cancer can become an overwhelming and central focus in patients' lives, and the issue is that for some cancers, it's actually not the thing that is most threatening to them," says Snyder. "Especially for things like early-stage breast cancer, patients are more likely to die of other things like heart disease."

Both Snyder and the IOM recommend that cancer specialists work with survivors' primary care providers to ensure that all health-care needs are met. "Non-cancer-related care is as important as cancer follow-up," says Snyder.

It's interesting that this phenomenon isn't the same for all cancer survivors. According to Snyder's research, breast cancer survivors are pretty good at going back to "routine medical care," while prostate cancer patients do better in some areas and worse in others. "But our unfortunate colorectal cancer survivors consistently compare worse to people who have never had colorectal cancer in terms of their co-morbid condition care," Snyder says. It is unclear why this is the case.

The key is to remember that the human body needs all kind of medical care, not just oncological care. Snyder's research says that the people who do the best in terms of overall health care are those who see both their cancer and primary care docs. So, even if you don't have a survivorship care plan, you can still follow this IOM recommendation: pull out your calendar and set up those appointments.

DIY: Journey Forward

If your doctors haven't offered you a survivorship care plan, there's a do-it-yourself version online. Journey Forward (www. journeyforward.org) provides a free, easy-to-use software program that helps you create a custom Survivorship Care Plan based on the surveillance guidelines developed by the American Society of Clinical Oncology (ASCO). It has been developed by several organizations, including the National Coalition for Cancer Survivorship, UCLA Cancer Survivorship Center, Genentech, and WellPoint, Inc. "It's a cool service," says Matasar.

The hope is that these survivorship care plans will help patients and their doctors (oncology team, primary care doctor, and other health-care professionals) coordinate post-treatment—maybe even coordinate it with electronic medical records—possibly even develop a national, unified, and consistent approach, without having people feel like Wile E. Coyote pedaling in mid-air.

Survivorship care plans are becoming more and more common. But, to my mind, this isn't happening quickly enough. Ask your oncology doctors for one. It will help guide you through your post-treatment life and, hopefully, encourage physicians to institutionalize the practice. Maybe you can help more than just yourself.

Frequently Asked Questions

Q: Why don't I have a survivorship care plan?

A: Not all doctors and hospitals offer them. Ask your favorite oncologist for a plan. The more patients who request a survivorship care plan, the more likely the profession is to institutionalize the practice.

Q: Who creates a survivorship plan?

A: Survivorship plans are relatively new. Ideally, the oncologist or health-care facility initiates the process.

Q: How do I find out how doctors should monitor me to make sure I don't have a recurrence?

A: A survivorship care plan outlines the future tests, scans, and examinations that doctors will conduct to check for any recurrence, spreading, or future cancers.

Q: Can I create my own survivorship care plan?

A: Journey Forward (www.journeyforward.org) offers a basic template that allows patients and their health-care providers to put together an individual survivorship care plan.

Chapter 12

Exercise

Tito was only a fifteen-year-old high schooler when he was diagnosed with Hodgkins Disease. He should have been focusing on his favorite activities: wrestling on the school team, weight lifting at the gym, and playing basketball, not going to doctor's appointments, getting blood work done, and receiving chemotherapy.

But there he was, a virile-looking cancer patient, if you can have such a thing. He experienced very few side effects of the cancer treatment, lucky guy. Tito's doctors told him to stop exercising, boxing, and lifting weights. It's the same mantra doctors had been saying to cancer patients for years: take it easy, rest, relax. Catch up on your reading or get a subscription to Netflix. Don't overdo it. Tito's doctors told him he would be vulnerable to injury during chemo and he could hurt himself by exercising. But that wasn't Tito's style.

"I was sort of a stubborn Hodgkins patient," says Tito. "I couldn't really deal with someone telling me not to do something. I did the opposite of what they told me." Instead of switching from the gym to the chemo suite, Tito did both. He actually did stop wrestling, but instead of putting down the weights, he started lifting more and more. "I was fighting cancer, and the gym was my battlefield," he explains.

Losing his hair didn't stop Tito. "People just thought I had shaved my head." Some of his friends shaved their heads in solidarity. It wasn't exactly a major public announcement, though; a group of African American teenagers with bald heads seemed more like a statement of fashion than of medical status. But it helped Tito feel like he wasn't alone in his cancer journey.

Tito's doctors weren't happy with his muscular approach, though. Looking at a chest scan one time, Tito's doctor noticed that he was gaining muscle. "You may want to ease back on that a little bit," Tito was told. He nodded politely.

But that wasn't the way Tito operated. "I hear stuff like that and I just push more," he says. Tito continued training, increasing his lifting weight bit by bit as he went through chemo.

Perhaps the most important muscle Tito honed was his mind. "I've learned that the mind is the most powerful tool you possess. If you believe it, it will happen," says Tito. Faith in God also played a role. "I really believe that if you believe, you just have to have faith. If you have doubts, that's when it starts to trick you," he explains. Tito had no doubts, neither in his physical prowess nor his faith.

After finishing cancer treatment, Tito became increasingly interested in weight lifting and starting living the bodybuilding lifestyle. He began reading muscle magazines, eating with discipline, and focusing on intense weightlifting. "Lifting weights was a great way to beat the stress associated with cancer," Tito says. "I always felt my best after a tough lifting session, so I began lifting regularly." Since then, Tito has become a competitive bodybuilder and has placed in more than a dozen bodybuilding tournaments. He never resorted to steroids and has been called "one of New York City's top natural bodybuilders."

Not only that, Tito works as a trainer, to help impart what he's learned about fitness and bodybuilding to others. "I loved the idea of helping others improve their physiques and their health," he says, and he particularly likes the idea that his cancer experience can help others. "My approach towards working with regular people is to expose them to health and wellness through diet and exercise. Not everyone wants to be a competitive bodybuilder," Tito admits. "But that doesn't mean that they can't use the strategies of the successful bodybuilder."

Yael sits—not stands—on the other end of the continuum. She'd always done some sort of exercise, but she treated it more like taking daily vitamins than anything she was particularly passionate about. It was good to do, nothing particularly fun, and if she missed a day, so be it. She had tried different things over the years, from weight training to yoga and from biking through the suburbs to taking aerobics classes in the city, but never found an activity that she really fell in love with.

Finally, after Yael had a lumpectomy, her second bout of cancer, she decided: enough is enough. She'd had tumors in different parts of her body and felt like she didn't know where cancer would pop up next. She needed to get her whole body in better shape.

She walked over to the gym just a few blocks from her house and joined. She thought about easing her way into it by taking a class or two, but she knew herself. "I take a class or two, start to worry about the cost, and promise myself I'll take a power walk in Central Park every other day instead," she says. "Then it rains or gets cold or hot and pretty soon I don't need to find an excuse. The question doesn't even arise anymore."

The gym works for Yael because it offers classes. In fact, she admits that she hasn't hit the weight room once. (OK, she did get the initial tour of the machines with a demonstration on how to use them, but, she says, "Honestly, I no longer remember which machines they showed me, much less what to do with or on them.") Instead Yael has been taking Zumba (for aerobic exercise) and Pilates (for strength).

Yael is in her mid-forties, so the advantage to Zumba is that "I'm usually the oldest person in the room. I could be the mother of most of the kids in there." That means she feels no competition. "As long as I remain upright, sweat, and don't cause any traffic accidents, I'm doing fine," she says. "Pilates is fun because, well, how much can you kvetch about an exercise class where you spend most of the time on your back?"

Tito Was Right

It turns out, though, that Tito was right. For years, doctors believed the advice they gave Tito: take it easy and let the treatment do its work. Recently, though, researchers have found that exercise is one of the few things people can do to decrease their chances of getting cancer, having a recurrence, or dying of cancer.

"Regular physical activity is good for everyone," says Jennifer Ligibel, MD, medical oncologist at Boston's Dana Farber Cancer Institute. "There is good evidence that exercise is especially helpful for cancer survivors, especially breast, colon, and prostate cancer." In fact, exercise can lower a woman's chances of being diagnosed with breast cancer by somewhere between 25 percent and 30 percent.

"Our physicians here are big proponents of exercise, and they believe that no matter what stage you are in, no matter what part of treatment you are in, beginning, middle, or end, you should exercise in order to deal with the consequences of the treatment—the fatigue, the lymphedema, all those issues that may occur due to treatment," says Daniel Destin, manager of Shipley Fitness Center at Newton-Wellesley Hospital in the western suburbs of Boston. Doctors at Newton-Wellesley Hospital, says Destin, find that cancer survivors who exercise have better outcomes and a better overall quality of life.

That doesn't mean exercise is entirely protective, of course. "Marathon runners get breast cancer, too," Ligibel says. But getting out there and exercising on a regular basis can really help. It's one of the few concrete things we can do to decrease our chances of recurrence. "The data are strongest for breast cancer, but exercise is helpful for all cancer survivors," the oncologist adds.

Weight Gain

Body weight is always, well, a weighty issue. Many people struggle with it, whether or not they've had cancer. When they're stressed, they eat; when they're worried, they eat; when they're concerned about their weight—you see where I'm going. Cancer doesn't help the situation.

When I was on chemotherapy, I gained thirty pounds. Along with my weight, my cholesterol went up. When I reached my "new normal," I lost it, every last ounce. People even told me I looked better than before I had cancer, which was nice to hear—as was the fact that my cholesterol level had dropped along with my weight. But then I was diagnosed with breast cancer, went on Tamoxifen (which I call chemo lite), and the numbers on the scale headed back up again.

Studies have shown—and I find this reassuring—that women who've been treated for breast cancer, especially those who have received chemotherapy treatment, are often overweight or obese. This is true for as much as three years after treatment is over.[1] Unfortunately, the researchers haven't figured out quite why this is the case, nor what to do about it.

Jennifer Merschdorf, breast cancer survivor and CEO of Young Survival Coalition (YSC), knows what I'm talking about. "I really struggle a lot with weight gain," she says, thanks to chemo-pause, otherwise known as chemically induced menopause. "Before cancer, I was really, really small," she says. And weight gain? "It's really hard, really hard stuff," she says.

1. Janet L. Espirito et al., "Bridging to Survivorship in Breast Cancer: Learning How Treatment Impacts Mental Health Among Early-State Breast Cancer Survivors," *Journal of Clinical Oncology* 31 (2013).

Lindsey agrees, too. "I haven't had a steady weight, a steady clothing size since" being diagnosed with leukemia a few years earlier. She gained about thirty pounds during her year on chemotherapy, then lost it all. At one point, she had hit 103 pounds, "and I looked very bony," she remembers. "Since then, I've been gaining and then I held steady for a while. But all I needed to do was have a lot of stress in my life and I gained fifteen pounds," says Lindsey. It has caused the thirty-three-year-old to lose confidence in her appearance, which is especially hard for a young, single woman.

Jennifer worries that doctors don't take the issue seriously enough. "I say this to doctors a lot, when I'm in meetings or wherever I am. Don't just say, 'It can cause weight gain,' in passing. Stop there. That is a *huge* deal," she adds. "It affects a person's psyche, it affects their checkbooks and their pocketbooks, it affects everything," she says. "It affects every aspect of their lives."

It's true for every person, every woman, of every age. It is, perhaps, even more difficult, though, for young women like Jennifer and Lindsey who've been thrust into early menopause because of their treatment, she points out. "Their peers are not going through that," says Jennifer. Most twenty- and thirty-somethings aren't experiencing the hot flashes, insomnia, and—let's not forget—weight gain that comes along with the end of menstruation and fertility. So when you're the only one you know struggling with weight issues, well, it makes the challenge even more difficult.

The Risks of Weight Gain

We've long known that being overweight or obese increases your chances of certain diseases, such as heart disease and diabetes. More recently, researchers have figured out that it also amplifies the possibility of getting cancer, especially for post-menopausal breast cancer and cancers of the colon and rectum, pancreas, kidney, esophagus, and endometrium, according to the American Cancer Society. If that isn't enough, obesity also raises the chances of mortality from cancer.

Perhaps more to the point, obesity is known to increase the chances of having a cancer recurrence, especially for women who've had breast cancer or men who have had prostate cancer.

The lines between underweight, normal weight, and overweight are pretty clear, thanks to work by the National Institutes of Health (NIH). NIH has determined that a person's healthy weight should relate to that person's height.[2] This holds true for Caucasians, African Americans, Latinos, and Native Americans, but Asians are an exception; they are at risk of obesity with lower weights.[3]

To help people figure out where they are on the normal to extremely obese continuum, NIH developed the Body Mass Index (BMI). If you look up your height and weight, you can see what your BMI is and plan accordingly. There's a copy of the chart in Appendix 2 (pages 295–296).

Exercise, though, is important for everyone—whether you're underweight, normal, or obese. We were designed to make fire, build structures, farm the land, and run away from scary beasts, not to sit around typing on a keyboard, driving a car, or talking into a small metal device. Just about every human body needs to get moving.

American Cancer Society Guidelines

How much exercise is good? Surely not every survivor needs to give Tito a run for his money, as it were.

Researchers and health-care experts have been talking about the importance of exercise for a long time. The American Cancer Society (ACS) had been publishing articles about the importance of physical activity for more than a decade. But the organization wasn't

2. "Assessing Your Weight and Health Risk," *National Institutes of Health*, accessed December 4, 2013, http://www.nhlbi.nih.gov/health/public/heart/obesity/lose_wt/risk.htm.

3. WHO Expert Consultation, "Appropriate body-mass index for Asian populations and its implications for policy and intervention strategies," *The Lancet* 363 (January 10, 2004): 157-63, http://www.ncbi.nlm.nih.gov/pubmed/14726171.

prepared to come right out and tell people to move their behinds to protect against cancer until 2012.

That year, the ACS issued its *Guidelines on Nutrition and Physical Activity for Cancer Prevention.* "Now the data are strong enough to call our recommendations 'Guidelines,'" says Colleen Doyle, MS, RD, Director of Nutrition and Physical Activity at the American Cancer Society. That may seem like a minor difference in word choice, but for the ACS it represents a huge change.

Basically, the guidelines are threefold:

1. Adults should exercise every week. It's best to spend at least an hour and a half on moderate-intensity activity, or an hour and a quarter on vigorous activity. The ACS recommends spreading this activity throughout the week. I find that living in a third-floor walk-up apartment guarantees that I do at least a little bit of stair climbing every day. It's not enough, but it's a start.

2. Children and adolescents should be even more active than their parents. The ACS recommends that young people spend at least an hour per day in moderate or vigorous intensity activity. They should aim for doing vigorous activity at least three days each week.

3. The flip side of increasing your activity is limiting sedentary behavior. The ACS recommends trying to spend less time sitting, lying down, watching television, or indulging in what I call "screen time." I've tried to convince my kids that this rule isn't mine, that it comes from the American Cancer Society, but they're not buying it.[4]

---

4. "American Cancer Society Guidelines on Nutrition and Physical Activity for Cancer Prevention," *American Cancer Society*, last modified January 11, 2012, http://www.cancer.org/healthy/eathealthygetactive/acsguidelinesonnutritionphysical activityforcancerprevention/acs-guidelines-on-nutrition-and-physical-activity-for-cancer-prevention-intro.

The point to remember is that doing something is always better than doing nothing. A little exercise is better than none; a lot is preferable to a little. Most of all, doing some physical activity above the usual activities, no matter what you do, can have many health benefits. Exercise is good for you whether or not you lose weight.

The ACS guidelines focus on aerobic exercise says Doyle, the ACS nutritionist, but that doesn't mean that strength and flexibility training are unimportant. (Yael will be relieved to hear that her weekly Pilates classes "count.") More people exercise by walking than in any other way, so that's why the ACS focuses on aerobic workouts. But strength-based exercise is important, too. In fact, weight training can help breast cancer survivors avoid lymphedema. The ACS recommends that people do a combination of aerobic and strength training to improve their chances of avoiding recurrence.

"The aerobic part you need for increased circulation. It can definitely make you feel better," says Destin, the fitness center manager. "You get more chemicals to the brain, more blood to the brain, higher amounts of energy," he adds.

But aerobics alone isn't enough. "Strength training is a good idea because during treatment, a lot of muscles atrophy, you get imbalances, and you might get joint pain," Destin says. The key, he says, "is to straighten up those core muscles to help mitigate lower back pain [and give you an] overall sense of feeling stronger."

Despite Yael's regimen, strength training is more than just Pilates, says Destin. Other effective ways to improve core strength are yoga, training with weights, and even using your own body weight. If you remember those push-ups and sit-ups from gym class, way back when, that stuff can be helpful now.

When to Begin, What to Do

Tito is a bit of an outlier. He was probably outdoing the ACS recommendations from the time he could toddle across the floor in a diaper. There's inspiration, and then there's intimidation; I know that if I felt like I had to keep up with Tito, I think I'd just throw in the towel, sit down on the sofa, and crack open a box of chocolate chip cookies. Fortunately, that's not the case. Exercise can improve your quality of life—and possibly lengthen it—but it needn't take over your life altogether.

Jennifer Merschdorf, who was diagnosed with breast cancer at age thirty-six and is now a survivor and CEO of Young Survival Coalition (YSC), is probably a better example of taking it step by step. Jennifer came to her post-treatment exercise regimen in a sort of sideways manner. She started at YSC just months after finishing her own treatment for breast cancer. That first year, she met a woman in her thirties who had metastatic breast cancer and had just completed the Tour de Pink, YSC's fundraising bike ride. Two hundred miles in three days—with metastatic cancer, no less. Wow, thought Jennifer. If she can do it, so can I. So, the next year, Jennifer signed up to participate.

The catch is that Jennifer hadn't gotten on a bicycle since she was about ten years old. She hated bikes. "Hated, hated, hated them," she emphasizes. Oh—and one more little detail: despite the cliché, Jennifer had, actually, forgotten how to ride a bike. "My husband had to teach me," she says. "I fell a lot, scraped my knees a lot."

Jennifer hadn't exactly been an exercise fanatic prior to diagnosis. "I never exercised before," she says. "I did it to prove that I could. I did it to prove that I'm alive and well." No one was convinced she would pull it off. "My husband and my brother didn't believe I would do it," she admits. "They 'fessed up later," after she had proven them wrong.

Following the YSC twelve-week training guide that culminates in the Tour de Pink, Jennifer started out biking an hour at a time, slowly building up her strength and stamina. The YSC regimen incorporates easy riding days, endurance riding days, and stretching days. She built up her pace and endurance bit by bit. "I trained my little butt off," she says. Her husband, an avid cyclist, trained with her.

Crossing the finish line was an amazing feeling for Jennifer. "I got it done," she says, with pride in her voice. "I did something that most of my friends can't do. Non-cancer people, perfectly happy, healthy people. Most people can't do it." It was a major accomplishment.

Jennifer didn't exactly lead the way. "I was dead last two days in a row," she says. "But my mom was always there just waiting for me." It wasn't about winning the race for Jennifer—it was about completing the challenge. "That was pretty big for me," she says. "It was powerful. Determination is a powerful thing."

As it turns out, the Tour de Pink wasn't a one-time thing for Jennifer. She's signed up to do it again, and now she and her husband exercise and bike together regularly. "I spend a lot of time on the bike now; it's fun," she says. In a weird way, what started out as a way for Jennifer to prove that she was alive and healthy, a survivor, has evolved into a strategy to help keep her that way.

Basically, you should start exercising as soon after treatment as you comfortably can. Don't shove your surgical drains in a pocket, lace up your sneakers, and go out for a ten-mile run; your body needs time to heal. Start by walking the hospital hallways, or make circles around your own living room. Maybe head out to get the mail. As you feel better, you can move on to bigger and better exercise. Studies show that exercise before treatment begins, during treatment, and after treatment, are all linked to a decrease in recurrence.

"Today is the best time to get started," says Ligibel, the medical oncologist at Dana Farber. It doesn't matter what you do, as long as you get your heart rate up and sweat a bit. But, of course, you should delay activity if you are anemic; wait until you get the all-clear from your doctor. Be careful where you go if you are in chemotherapy and have a low white blood cell count or if you have had a bone marrow transplant, as you will be more susceptible to catching an infection.

"The message is that the amount and type of exercise you do should be based on how active you were before you were diagnosed and what type of cancer and treatment you've experienced," says

Doyle at the American Cancer Society. Talk to your doctors, she proposes, for a sort of "exercise prescription."

Ligibel says that most people choose to walk, at a moderate pace. That means about a twenty-minute mile—not speed walking by any stretch, but you want to try to do better than toddler speed.

For someone who's not active at all, Ligibel recommends starting with walking about ten minutes a day a couple of times a week and working up from there. Anything extra that you do puts you ahead of where you were before you started. "It is important to set realistic goals," says Ligibel. She proposes trying for ten thousand steps a day, as counted by a pedometer.

Try to fit it into your daily life. Get off the subway a stop or two early, park your car at the far end of the parking lot, or ditch mechanized transit altogether and try just walking or biking. If you do it on the way to work or to an appointment, the need to arrive on time will guarantee that you reach the recommended moderate pace.

Newton-Wellesley's Program

Not everyone is lucky enough to have a program such as that at Newton-Wellesley Hospital, located in the Boston suburbs. There, patients are sent to the Shipley Fitness Center by their doctors. "Exercise is medicine for them," Destin, the center manager explains.

Destin starts by conducting an assessment of the person. "We look at range of motion; we talk about any joint issues they may have, any orthopedic issues or co-morbidities," he explains. Destin also asks about the person's goals. "One woman just wanted to be able to vacuum her apartment by herself." When he understands the person's goals and limitations, he designs an individualized exercise program. Survivors meet with a trainer regularly.

The key, Destin finds, is pinpointing the right program for the individual. It's not just a matter of determining how much aerobic exercise is appropriate and what muscles to strengthen. "We have to find out what motivates people to come in," he says. "We can't just give them a general exercise program. If they don't like it, they won't do it. We really sit down and we go over exercises."

That means that if the person likes a particular exercise, Destin encourages it, but if not, he searches for a substitute. "If they don't like the treadmill, we'll introduce the elliptical. If they don't like spring training on the machines, we'll do some body weight exercises on the floor. If they don't like the floor, we have a little table that they can use instead," says Destin. "We really try to accommodate them and their needs, make them comfortable, keep them comfortable." Working with the person improves the chances of success, he has found.

If you're doing it solo, then, remember that you're more likely to stick with an activity you enjoy. Chocolate beats out medicine. And if that means, like Yael found, that you have to switch your exercise routine every so often, so be it. You're not aiming to be an Olympic swimmer or runner; you just want to be around to watch the next Olympics on TV.

Exercising after cancer isn't exactly the same as exercising after some other illness or injury, says Destin. "If you look at post-menopausal women, after treatment, they have a higher incidence of fractures; they're weaker. So you have to be aware of that," says Destin.

It's not just women. "Post-chemotherapy you have to watch out for neuropathies in their hands and feet, so you have to tailor your exercises accordingly," the trainer explains. "If they have it in their feet, you have to try to strengthen the muscles on the lower leg so they can keep their balance. If they have some in the hands, you want to strengthen the forearm muscles as much as possible to improve their grip." Exercise doesn't necessarily prevent neuropathy, Destin emphasizes. But it can help you cope with it.

Finding a Trained Trainer

Exercise is not a one-size-fits all recipe. Different types of cancer require varying treatments, and these treatments affect the body in various ways. And, of course, these diverse side effects demand their own distinct sorts of activities to strengthen the body and get it back to "normal."

That's why it can also be helpful to work with a trainer who knows about cancer survivorship. There are several programs out there offering these specialized services. The Livestrong Foundation, working with a large number of local YMCA branches, has developed a twelve-week, small-group program designed for adult cancer survivors; it offers emotional support as well as training advice. (See Appendix 1: Resources for Survivorship for more information.)

Another option is to check the trainer's credentials. The American College of Sports Medicine, together with the ACS, offers a training certification that teaches people how to design and administer fitness assessments and exercise programs specific to a client's cancer diagnosis, treatment, and current recovery status.[5] Daniel Destin is one of the first graduates of this program.

Exercise as a Place of Peace

When Joe was in high school, he'd been on the basketball team and had exercised regularly. But when he went to college, he got busy with academics, and exercise fell by the wayside. "I gained almost fifty pounds in a semester and a half," he remembers. "That was obviously problematic." Then he was diagnosed with non-Hodgkin's lymphoma.

It took a couple of years after he finished cancer treatment to get back to his exercise routine. In 2002, he prepared to participate in a Team in Training one-hundred-mile bike ride around Lake Tahoe. Team in Training is a fundraising project of the Leukemia and Lymphoma Society. It became a regular part of his life. "Now I'm a huge cyclist; it's kind of a constant in my life," Joe says. He also plays basketball a few times a week.

---

5. "ACSM/ACS Certified Cancer Exercise/TrainerSM," *American College of Sports Medicine*, accessed December 5, 2013, http://certification.acsm.org/acsm-cancer-exercise-trainer.

Joe's goal was to keep in good shape—and avoid the fifty pounds he gained when he stopped exercising in college. But more than that, exercise functions almost like meditation for Joe.

"I consider the bike my church," Joe says. "It's where I go to kind of zone out and think about life." Joe is a small business owner and is married with a preschool daughter—plenty to keep him busy. Biking is for Joe as meditation or yoga is for other people. "It's peaceful," he says.

Many Benefits

Exercise can bring you peace and can help prevent cancer recurrence. But it does more than that. It also builds muscle strength, bone health, and endurance, according to Doyle. And, of course, it lowers the risk of diabetes, heart disease, arthritis, depression, and other diseases and conditions.

Exercise can improve your quality of life. It often decreases stress and anxiety and boosts self-esteem. It can raise your energy level, enhance your mood, and help control your weight. Not only that, it often makes you sleep better and even improves your sex life. Yael realized she likes a few types of exercise. Jennifer found that her newfound interest in biking gave her and her husband an activity to enjoy together. And, of course, Tito found that exercise provided him with a profession and a wall full of bodybuilder awards.

Frequently Asked Questions

Q: When should cancer survivors return to exercise?

A: Immediately. Talk to your health-care provider about what sort of activity is good for you, but it's always good to start doing something as soon as you feel able.

Q: But I thought I was supposed to take it easy and let my body heal. Shouldn't I just rest after treatment?

A: We keep learning more and more about health care. Scientific research indicates that cancer survivors benefit from exercise. It can decrease chances of a recurrence or new cancer by a good percentage.

Q: Should I do aerobic exercise, or should I stick with strength training?

A: Both are useful for cancer survivors. The best option would be a combination of the two.

Q: How do I find a trainer who knows about my needs as a cancer survivor?

A: Both the Livestrong Foundation and the American College of Sports Medicine, together with the American Cancer Society (ACS) teaches exercise trainers about the special needs of cancer survivors. Check credentials if you're looking for trainers with special education.

Chapter 13

Nutrition

After she finished treatment for breast cancer, Deni wanted to do something to cut her chances of recurrence or getting a new cancer. She did a lot of research and decided to focus on nutrition. "Obviously I wanted to live," says Deni, breast cancer survivor. So she changed her eating habits dramatically.

"I cut out all sodas, all candies, anything sweet," she says. This was a challenge for Deni, especially because friends and family members kept bringing her cookies and muffins, no matter how many times she asked them not to. But Deni understood why they did. "Food is how you show love, right?" Deni notes. But that didn't mean she had to eat it all, though once it was sitting in her kitchen, staring at her, it was hard to say no.

In addition to eliminating sugar, Deni also stopped eating soy products, unfiltered tap water, and most foods that aren't organic. She drinks a lot less and has quit smoking. Deni doesn't buy everything organic; some items are just too expensive. "If I don't buy organic, I buy minimally treated," she says. "That means that while they use some pesticides, they don't use that much."

To boost her vegetable consumption, Deni joined the Park Slope Food Co-op as well as a Community Supported Agriculture (CSA) group. She even tried growing her own tomatoes, but "that didn't work out so well," Deni explains. Gardening can be difficult when you live in New York City.

The co-op sells local and organic produce, pasture-raised and grass-fed meat, free-range, organic poultry, wild and sustainably farmed fish, and a host of other products. They even have environmentally safe cleaning supplies. "I do most of my shopping there," Deni says.

She enjoyed the CSA, too, for a while, along with a group of neighbors. For an initial investment in a local organic farmer's business, she got weekly deliveries of organic vegetables, mostly greens, a big cardboard box stuffed with lettuce, kale, Swiss chard, mustard greens, or collard greens. Plus a smattering of tomatoes, cucumbers, a variety of squash, strawberries, green beans, peppers, onions, garlic, and garlic scapes.

"It was great and very reasonably priced," she remembers. "But then the farmer decided he wasn't making enough money to justify driving into the city every week," says Deni. Such are the challenges of living in the city. So now she's back to shopping mostly at the co-op.

Deni switched to organic food for several reasons. She wanted to avoid the pesticides and herbicides that get added to plants and the hormones and antibiotics that are often found in conventionally grown livestock. She figured she'd consumed enough foreign substances between chemotherapy and her several surgeries. Deni had had a few lumpectomies before her mastectomy.

Not only that, Deni didn't want to take the hormone treatments that were recommended to prevent recurrence. She tried Tamoxifen for a while, decided that the side effects were too difficult to live with. "So that's the other reason I eat organic," Deni explains—to try to protect her body from recurrence.

Not that Deni's eating habits are perfect. "I still eat too many cookies, too much ice cream," she says. "Sometimes I eat organic cookies. But sometimes I don't," she admits. "Sometimes I just walk right down to the corner store and get those Pepperidge Farm cookies." Not surprisingly, she tends to increase her sugar intake just before her oncologist appointments. Worry will do that.

Since Deni switched to organic food, she's seen some real health improvements. She hasn't had a cold in five years, and her allergies are much better. "I'm allergic to nature," she explains. Symptoms hit her in the spring and fall when the pollen counts rise. Of course, she does take other precautions. "During allergy season, I avoid milk, nuts, and alcohol because all those things are irritants to me," she says. It works for her.

Veggies Are the Way to Go

We don't yet know everything there is to know about nutrition and cancer prevention. But researchers have come up with some basic rules. The most basic, according to the American Institute for Cancer Research (AICR), involves simple division: fill up your plate with two-thirds plant foods and one-third animal protein—which supports Deni's approach.[1]

When the AICR mentions plant foods, it's talking about vegetables, fruits, whole grains, and beans, preferably the more colorful variety. Dark leafy greens, tomatoes, strawberries, blueberries, carrots, and cantaloupe are especially rich in vitamins, minerals, and the phytochemicals that can reduce cancer risk.

When it comes to animal proteins, its best to stick with fish, poultry, lean red meat, and cheese, and limit consumption of processed meats such as cold cuts, bacon, sausage, and ham.

Watch out for snacking. It's not necessarily bad; it all depends on what you munch on. Hitting the vending machines at work probably means you'll get more sodium, sugar, cholesterol, and trans fats than if you bring a bag of carrot sticks, an apple, dried seaweed, or some other healthier option from home. If you're looking to satisfy your

---

1. "Foods That Fight Cancer," *American Institute for Cancer Research*, accessed December 4, 2013, http://www.aicr.org/foods-that-fight-cancer/.

sweet tooth, nutritionists recommend trying less familiar fruits, such as kiwi and papaya. I know I've gotten hooked on dried mango (without added sugar).

It's also helpful to watch how much you eat of certain items:

- **Sodium.** A sneaky little condiment, sodium hides in most processed foods, so read those labels carefully. It's best to have fewer than 2,300 milligrams a day, though African Americans, people over age fifty-one, and anyone with hypertension, diabetes, or chronic kidney disease should have even less; they should shoot for a maximum of 1,500 milligrams per day. Nutritionists recommend substituting herbs and spices such as basil, turmeric, paprika, thyme, and dill for added flavor.
- **Alcohol.** Try to have no more than one drink a day for women and two a day for men
- **Tobacco.** This is one item to cut out entirely. No smoking, no chewing tobacco.
- **Sugary drinks and foods.** Processed foods that are high in fat or in added sugar or are low in fiber have little to offer a healthy diet. The calories are pretty much empty of nutritional benefit.
- **Saturated fatty acids.** Limit them to less than 10 percent of your daily calories and replace with mono-saturated and polyunsaturated fatty acids.
- **Cholesterol.** Try to consume fewer than 300 milligrams per day of dietary cholesterol.
- **Trans fatty acid.** Limit foods that contain synthetic sources of trans fats (such as partially hydrogenated oils) and other solid fats.
- **Refined grains.** Watch these, too, especially refined grain foods that contain solid fats, added sugars, and sodium.[2]

---

2. "American Cancer Society Guidelines on Nutrition and Physical Activity for Cancer Prevention," *American Cancer Society*, last modified January 11, 2013, http:// www.cancer.org/healthy/eathealthygetactive/acsguidelinesonnutritionphysical activityforcancerprevention/acs-guidelines-on-nutrition-and-physical-activity-for-cancer-prevention-intro.

While you're tweaking your diet, it's helpful to increase the "good stuff" as well as limit the bad. Specifically, the AICR recommends adding these food items to your diet:

- **Vegetables and fruit.** Focus on dark green, red, and orange vegetables as well as beans and peas.
- **Whole grains.** Try to make at least half of the grains you eat be whole grains, and get rid of those refined grains.
- **Fat-free or low-fat milk and milk products.** This includes yogurt, cheese, and fortified soy beverages.
- **Varied protein.** Include seafood, lean meat, and poultry, eggs, beans and peas, soy products, and nuts and seeds. Opt for unsalted nuts and seeds to cut your sodium intake, but remember, these yummy treats often carry a high caloric price tag.
- **Seafood.** It's better for you than meat and poultry, says the AICR.
- **Oils.** They're healthier than solid fats.

Some people rely on vitamin and mineral supplements to get in all the nutrients they need. Unfortunately, convenient as they are, pills aren't as effective as actual food. The body absorbs the good stuff more readily from food than from supplements. But if you're just not getting enough from food alone, no matter how hard you try, pills might just do the trick.

Phytochemicals

Phytochemicals are naturally occurring chemicals in plants. "Phyto" means "plant" in Greek. These chemicals provide the plants with their color, odor, and flavor. They're even more helpful with humans, though they don't turn us deep red or green. Rather, according to the AICR, phytochemicals

- Stimulate the immune system

- Keep the substances we eat, drink, and breathe from becoming carcinogenic
- Decrease the sort of inflammation and oxidative damage that makes cancer growth more likely
- Prevent DNA damage and help with DNA repair
- Slow the growth rate of cancer cells
- Encourage damaged cells to commit suicide before they can reproduce
- Help regulate hormones[3]

See Appendix 3 for more detailed information on which phytochemicals appear in which foods, and what the benefits of each are.

The Joy of Soy

There's been a lot of controversy over whether women who've had breast cancer can eat soy. After years of research, the AICR has determined that, in fact, soy is perfectly safe for breast cancer survivors, eaten in moderation. For people who've had other types of cancer, soy foods do not increase risk; sometimes they can even lower risk of recurrence.

"Determining whether it is safe for breast cancer survivors to eat soy has been one of the big research questions under study, and now we know it is safe—the evidence is so consistent," said AICR nutrition advisor Karen Collins, MS, RD, CDN, an expert on diet and cancer prevention.[4]

Researchers had been concerned about isoflavones, a group of compounds present in soy that, in some ways, mimic the action of

---

3. "Phytochemicals: The Cancer Fighters in the Foods We Eat," *American Institute for Cancer Research*, April 10, 2013, http://www.aicr.org/reduce-your-cancer-risk/diet/elements_phytochemicals.html.

4. "Soy is Safe for Breast Cancer Survivors," *American Institute for Cancer Research*, February 4, 2013, http://www.aicr.org/cancer-research-update/2012/november_21_2012/cru-soy-safe.html.

estrogen. Studies of lab rats found that high blood levels of estrogen are linked to increased breast cancer risk, according to AICR. But it turns out that laboratory animals metabolize soy isoflavones differently than human beings do.

More to the point, the researchers say, soy doesn't increase our estrogen levels—and consuming moderate amounts of soy foods does *not* increase a breast cancer survivor's risk of recurrence or death. To clarify, when the AICR says a "moderate amount," it is referring to one or two servings per day; some studies suggest that three servings per day is safe, too.[5]

Soy doesn't decrease the risk of recurrence, at least as far as we know now. But for breast cancer survivors who are lactose intolerant and enjoy soy milk, those who are opting for more of a plant-based diet, or those who find it helpful in maintaining their weight, it's nice to know that soy is safe.

How About Grilling Out?

It just isn't summer without a little beach, sunburn, and barbecue. OK, so maybe you can skip the sunburn—but what's a summer without heating up the outdoor grill?

It is true that cooking beef, poultry, and fish under high heat isn't great for you; it can cause certain compounds to form—specifically hetero-cyclic amines (HCAs) and polycyclic aromatic hydrocarbons (PAHs)—and these compounds can change DNA to make it more hospitable to cancer growth. Smoke doesn't help, either, says the AICR. But you can keep on grilling if you follow these guidelines, suggests the AICR:

- **Watch what you grill.** Processed meats as well as beef, pork, and lamb aren't ideal for cancer survivors, no matter how

---

5. "Soy is Safe for Breast Cancer Survivors," *American Institute for Cancer Research*, www.aicr.org/press/press-releases/soy-safe-breast-cancer-survivors.html.

you prepare them. So try grilling fish and chicken. Consider using vegetables for a little variety; grilling brings out their sweetness.

- **Marinate.** For reasons that researchers haven't yet pinpointed, steeping meat, poultry, and fish for at least a half hour can reduce formation of those nasty HCAs. Inexplicably, it's particularly helpful to use a mixture of vinegar, lemon juice, or wine along with herbs and spices.

- **Preheat.** Because smoke exposure causes PAHs to form, it helps to cook the meat first. You can use a microwave, oven, or stove before you stick it on the grill. Any way you do it, the food spends less time on the grill—and you end up with a smaller amount of PAHs.

- **Use a low flame.** By keeping burning and charring to a minimum, less PAHs form on the meat. To reduce flare-ups, cut any visible fat off the meat, move coals to the side of the grill, and cook your meat in the center of the grill. Also, suggests the AICR, trim any charred portions before serving.[6]

Maintaining a Healthy Weight

As we saw in the chapter on exercise, maintaining a healthy weight is an important part of trying to prevent recurrence, according to the American Cancer Society, especially for women who have had breast cancer or men who have had prostate cancer. The National Institutes of Health (NIH) has developed a Body Mass Index chart (see Appendix 2) that can help you figure out your ideal weight.

Carrying extra body fat, especially around the abdomen, increases cancer risk, says the NIH. So, for people who have a high BMI, the

---

6. "Cancer Experts Issue '5-Steps' Warning on Grilling Safety," *American Institute for Cancer Research*, May 6, 2013, http://www.aicr.org/press/press-releases/5-steps-warning-grilling-safety.html.

simplified version of the plan is as follows: eat a little less; move a little more. Stick with foods that are lower in calories, notably vegetables, fruits, whole grains, and beans.

If you're underweight, the ACIR recommends two approaches: try milkshakes and smoothies made in a blender, or liquid commercial nutritional products. Some people also find that eating small, frequent meals throughout the day is easier on the stomach than having a large meal all at once. But just because you're underweight doesn't get you off the hook—you still need to exercise.

Choosing Healthy Foods

Is Deni right to avoid genetically modified organisms (GMOs) in our food? There's been no empirical evidence that GMOs are particularly problematic for cancer survivors. By the same token, no one's coming out and saying that they're good for us. But lots of people, including Deni, are leery of them.

Basically, genetically modified organisms are plants or animals that have been changed using genetic engineering with DNA from bacteria, viruses, or other plants or animals. GMOs exist in a form that is not available in nature, according to the Non-GMO Project.[7] Almost all GMOs have been developed to withstand the application of herbicides or insecticides. In other words, they are engineered to be invincible.

But they don't necessarily make us invincible. Specifically, people worry that GMOs can introduce allergens and toxins into our food, increase antibiotic resistance (especially with animal products), and create other environmental risks. In addition, certain organic fruits offer more vitamins and nutrients than their conventionally grown peers. As a result, more and more people are choosing organic fruits and vegetables to avoid exposure to many insecticides and herbicides.

---

7. "What is GMO?" *Non-GMO Project*, accessed December 4, 2013, http://www. nongmoproject.org/learn-more/what-is-gmo/.

Corn was one of the first crops to be grown widely using organophosphate, a broad-spectrum herbicide. These days, about 73 percent of US corn is genetically modified. We're not just talking about a side dish at the summer barbecue; corn is an ingredient in about three thousand products, including ethanol, cosmetics, ink, glue, laundry starch, medicines, and fabrics.

GMOs enter into other foodstuffs as well. Consider milk. Many dairy farmers use a genetically engineered "recombinant" version of the protein hormone called rBGH. The hormone increases milk production, but it also boosts the risk of clinical mastitis, which means more pus in the milk. It also leads to more use of antibiotics.

Many dairy farmers use antibiotics prophylactically, just in case, rather than wait for a cow to become ill. While this is probably easier for farmers, it can be harder on the rest of us. Researchers worry that these extra antibiotics play into the growth of antibiotic-resistant bacteria. The use of antibiotics can also cause elevated concentrations of insulin-like growth factor 1 (IGF-1), which has been positively associated with breast cancer risk.[8] Organic milk offers less hormones, antibiotics, and pus.

Now, for meat. It's not just dairy cows that get "extra" hormones and antibiotics. The beef industry, too, uses a variety of natural and synthetic hormones as well as a steady diet of low-dose antibiotics to increase beef production. Again, this likely contributes to the growth of antibiotic-resistant bacteria. Also, watch out for processed meats; the industry uses nitrates widely as preservatives in hot dogs, and nitrates have been linked to cancer.

Typically, US beef and poultry is irradiated to keep it from spoiling and to eliminate pathogens such as E. coli and Salmonella; this, too,

---

8. G. Fürstenberger and H. J. Senn, "Insulin-Like Growth Factors and Cancer," *Lancet Oncology* 3 (2002): 298–302.

carries risk for humans. Grass-fed beef not only lacks hormones and radiation; it has also been shown to contain more antioxidant vitamins and high levels of beneficial CLA.[9]

Shopping this way can be hard work. Juggling prices and family taste preferences is hard enough. It has been estimated that as much as 60 percent of the shelves in the typical supermarket are filled with foods containing GMOs. Eating GMO-free takes some careful label reading. Food co-ops, community-supported agriculture programs (CSAs), and farmers' markets can make it easier, though.

Eating organic should become even less difficult in the future. As consumers become more and more aware of the benefits of organic foods, they are much easier to find, in organic stores, food co-ops, and even a lot of standard supermarkets.

The truth of the matter is that there hasn't been a lot of research on the relationship between organic food and cancer survivors specifically. But studies have shown that avoiding GMOs is healthier for people in general—and cancer survivors deserve all the health perks they can get. Nutrition is a way that survivors can actively improve our health. Start with a plant-based diet, preferably organically grown plants, and add other protein sources. Watch your consumption of artificial additives and processed meats. And try to keep a healthy body weight. Easy peasy, huh?

Frequently Asked Questions:

Q: Do I have to become a vegetarian to prevent recurrence? Can't I have a hamburger once in a while?

A: The AICR recommends filling your plate with two-thirds fruits and vegetables and one-third animal protein. So hamburgers are fine, in moderation. Just don't fill up on them.

---

9. Cynthia A. Daley et al., "A Review of Fatty Acid Profiles and Antioxidant Content in Grass-Fed and Grain-Fed Beef," *Nutrition Journal* (2010): 1–12. doi:10.1186/1475-2891-9-10.

Q: What should I avoid to prevent cancer from coming back?

A: The AICR recommends watching your intake of sodium, alcohol, tobacco, sugar, saturated fatty acids, cholesterol, trans fats, and refined grains. Remember, there's no guarantee.

Q: What can I eat to decrease the chances of recurrence or a new cancer?

A: It can help to increase the amount of fruits, vegetables, fat-free or low-fat dairy, seafood, and oils, according to the AICR.

Q: What about soy? I've read so much about how it's not safe for breast cancer survivors.

A: There's been a lot of controversy on the topic, but the gavel is down—at least for now—and nutritionists agree that soy is safe, in moderation, for breast cancer survivors.

Q: How about grilling? Summer is prime time for barbecue. But is it safe for me to eat?

A: Grilling, like many other things, is OK in moderation. Try to marinate, shorten the grilling time, and consider including grilled vegetables in the mix.

Q: Does it help to eat organic?

A: Organic food often has more vitamins and nutrients than conventionally grown food does. In addition, it is usually free of pesticides, herbicides, hormones, and antibiotics. While most of the research doesn't focus on cancer survivors specifically, it has been shown to be healthier in general.

Chapter 14

East Asian Medicine

After I finished treatment for my third round of cancer, I figured it was time to try East Asian medicine (also known as Asian medicine). I couldn't decide if it was a matter of three strikes and you're out, or third time's a charm. Either way, I felt like I needed to try something new. I didn't realize how much there was to learn, though.

East Asian practitioners treat the whole body—body, mind, and soul. They focus not only on symptoms—in my case, low energy and depression—but also on lifestyle, emotional state, and overall health. It's a whole medical system, not just one or two modalities, though you don't have to do everything to reap some of the benefits.

I knew that acupuncture could increase energy, but I heard an amazing story from East Asian practitioner Ailin Kojima that really caught my attention. She told me about a man who had finished treatment for terminal prostate cancer and came to her for palliative care. "It was a quality of life issue for him," she explains. He was having difficulty eating and sleeping, he was cranky and moody, and he couldn't leave his apartment on his own.

He had one treatment, says Ailin, and was able to go home and take his dog out for a walk. He began to sleep better and to eat again too, which also helped his energy level. "It completely altered his mood to know that he could actually be happy about something, have some joy about something. He loved his dog very much. It really turned things around for him to be able to take his dog out," Ailin says. "He was really bitter and angry, and he kind of let go of that anger and was able to process through it and kind of make peace with his life before he died," she adds.

So I made an appointment with Michael Ishii, LAc, an East Asian practitioner who came recommended to me. Ishii is a New York state–licensed acupuncturist, a national board certified herbalist, and an East Asian dietary specialist, and is certified in medical qigong and kyoung therapy, which is Korean traditional osteopathic medicine. The initial consult, I was told, would last about two hours, about the amount of time I typically spend in a doctor's waiting room—except this time I'd spend that time with a practitioner instead of a good book.

After I chronicled my medical history, Ishii inspected my tongue, top and bottom. "The tongue is like a dipstick in the car," he says. "It's the only muscle that we can see internally that basically is submerged in the body fluids all the time," he explains. "It therefore reflects the electrolytic balance of fluids in the body and fluid metabolism." Then I jumped up on the table. Ishii palpated my middle and joints, then checked my pulse at my wrists. Apparently, my pulse reveals more to Ishii than to my internist; he gained information about all of my internal organs, not just my heart rate.

We also discussed nutrition. East Asian medicine emphasizes what goes into the body, and how it comes out. In many ways, it is not so different from Western medicine. Specifically, within East Asian medicine, there's an emphasis on eating small, regular meals, having a diversity of fruits and vegetables, and eating warm foods at every meal. Herbs are often important as are probiotics.

As he checked me, Ishii was exploring where, why, and how my qi became blocked. It turned out that my qi was depleted.

Chemotherapy, radiation, and surgery—not to mention daily living—will do that to you. The symptoms I described in my medical history were consistent with what Ishii found in his examination. "That's a good thing," Ishii said. "It's a more complicated situation when it's not consistent."

Then it was time for what Ishii called "needling." Ishii palpated the spot to find the precise location, called an acupoint, then he inserted the needle. Typically, acupuncturists use ten to twenty needles in a session. That's not quite the porcupine effect I had anticipated. I expected to feel a sensation somewhere between a pinprick and a hypodermic needle jab, and that probably does capture the initial feeling.

In a flash, the feeling changed. The sensation shot off in some direction. When he inserted a needle in my ankle, the sensation felt like a blob that turned into a stream and moved upward; when the needle went in by my knees, it shot downward; and when the needle went into my wrist, the sensation moved toward my finger tips. Incidentally, on my second treatment, the "blob" sensation disappeared, and each acupuncture insertion felt more like a single point of sensation that then moved up or down my body. Ishii always asked me which direction it moved in. "Sometimes the qi gets confused and goes the wrong way," he explains. "Then we must guide it back." I know the feeling; I get lost a lot myself.

Acupuncture is bilateral, so whenever Ishii put a needle in, say, one arm, he put another in the other arm at the same spot. Ishii was getting my sluggish qi moving, and the qi followed along the body's channels, called meridians.

I understand that there are thirty-six techniques used with insertion of the needles. But, honestly, I couldn't tell the difference, except for one time. Apparently my qi was particularly blocked in my left knee, so Ishii administered a little bit "extra" of his own qi along with the needle, which he called a coursing technique. I felt the needle insert in my knee, then a jolt of sensation in my ankle, with no sense of flowing in between. Clearly Ishii's qi moves faster than mine.

I lay there, with eight needles sticking out of me, for about five more minutes, which was very relaxing. The acupuncturist took my pulse again. "It's changed," he told me. "Now we have revealed what lies beneath all the stress and accumulation; I can tell how very, very exhausted you are."

East Asian medicine is a complex system—or a multiplicity of systems, across countries and lineages—that use four approaches or "pillars" to heal the human body, mind, and soul.

It is probably inappropriate to think about East Asian medicine by comparing it to the Western system of medicine, but it seems to be the only way I can wrap my Western-raised brain around the Eastern approach.

Incidentally, East Asian medicine is the longest surviving traditional system of medicine. It started a few thousand years ago in China, then spread to what is now Taiwan, Korea, and Japan. Lots of different variations arose, in various locations. The Communist government of China codified the system, removed all references to Daoism and Buddhism, and called it traditional Chinese medicine. TCM, as it is known, is probably the most well-known form of Chinese medicine in the West.

Western medicine calls lumps of cancer "tumors." East Asian medicine calls them "masses." (OK, they probably use some non-English term.) Western medicine uses four basic "hammers" (if you will) to treat these tumors: chemotherapy, surgery, radiation, and hormone therapy. East Asian medicine uses four approaches also, but they are different: acupuncture and moxibustion, diet and herbs, qigong, and physical manipulation. TCM practitioners tend not to use physical manipulation with cancer patients and survivors; it is not as effective with us as other techniques.

Perhaps the biggest difference between Western and East Asian medicine, as far as I can tell, is that Western medicine diagnoses and treats cancer, while East Asian medicine, greatly because of licensing and cultural issues, addresses the short- and long-term side effects of that Western treatment. Usually East Asian medicine helps patients get through treatment (dealing with nausea, fatigue, ad infinitum) and regain their strength once treatment is finished. In China, doctors use both East Asian and Western medicine to treat cancer; both medical approaches are equal partners.

As Ishii says, "From an East Asian medical perspective, when you arrive at the situation where you say you have cancer, there's a long road that led to that," he says. "It's not like you woke up suddenly and you had cancer." Instead, it's a little more complicated, just as in Western medicine. "There's a long road metabolically and having to do also with your environment and your constitution that led you down that road. And this is the stop you're at now."

The Human Body as Engine

If you remember back to your elementary school biology classes, Western medicine sees every organ as having a particular role. The heart pumps the blood. The lungs bring oxygen into the body and remove carbon dioxide. The kidneys filter the blood. These body parts all belong to various bodily systems: the circulatory system, the digestive system, the muscular system, and so on.

Eastern medicine also views our bodies as machines, though it looks at these machines through a slightly different lens.

First, there is qi, which is often translated from the Chinese as "energy," though from everything I hear and read, this translation doesn't really get at the full meaning of the term. "Qi is everything seen and unseen in our existence," Ishii says. "It's the building block of existence. For medical purposes, qi is the force of your metabolism," he says. "It's why you expire and exhale, it's why your heart pumps, it's why your pores open and close, it's the light in your eyes. Qi is also love." In other words, qi is a tad more than just energy.

Qi also governs what Western medicine calls homeostasis, which is often defined as a relatively stable equilibrium among various systems and parts. When qi is flowing properly in the body, all is well. When it isn't, well, it's time to go see an Eastern medical practitioner. "For example, when someone has road rage, that's an extreme manifestation of liver qi stagnation," says Ishii.

Ailin Kojima suggests that we think about qi as a sort of savings account. "You're given a lump sum of qi when you're born," she says, and it pretty much has to last you the rest of your life. "You can put a little bit of qi into your savings account during your lifetime," she says. You make withdrawals when you experience some trauma, either to the body or to the psyche. "But generally the withdrawals occur a lot more often" than the deposits. I don't know about you, but that's pretty much how my own bank account works. "When you start withdrawing too much," she says, "then you're really depleting yourself."

Typically, there are two types of Eastern medical practitioners: acupuncturists and herbalists, though in the United States many licensed practitioners do both. But you should check that out. Much as a radiation oncologist won't perform a hysterectomy and a medical oncologist relies on someone else to read and interpret X-rays, CT scans, and mammograms, many acupuncturists don't know about herbs. And vice versa. Be sure to see a practitioner who is licensed in acupuncture and has NCCAOM national herbal certification.

Sometimes, in extreme cases, practitioners will give some of their own qi to their patients. "We try to avoid that," says Kojima. "We're actually trained to do that only in very serious situations," she says. Instead, they try to add qi to their patients from elsewhere. "We have to work hard to make sure that we actually are extracting qi from the universe so that we are infusing our patients with that qi instead of giving up our own," she says—sort of like a qi conduit.

What Leads to Cancer

In Western medicine, health-care providers focus on the original site of the cancer. Lung cancer behaves differently than brain cancer does, which acts differently than leukemia does. If cancer metastasizes, it retains the qualities of its original form; we speak about, for instance, breast cancer that has spread to the lungs. The treatment protocols vary accordingly.

Eastern practitioners are concerned both with where the mass is located and with the underlying problems that led to its formation. I don't mean the cause; East Asian medicine doesn't know any more than Western medicine does about what is a stress-induced tumor and what is, say, caused by exposure to asbestos or radioactivity.

"Whenever there's a diagnosis of cancer, there's a qi weakness there," explains Ishii. In the East Asian medical system, practitioners figure that the body wasn't handling environmental forces effectively; the body's systems had some sorts of weaknesses. "And those deficiencies created some issues that were present along with the deficiency of the yuan qi," or source qi.

Kojima agrees. "We really want the qi to be flowing freely at all times," she says. "Because any time the qi flow is impeded, that creates an accumulation." Accumulations vary in size, she explains. Edema, for instance, is a relatively minor accumulation. Cancerous tumors on the other hand are, shall we say, a little more concerning. "Tumors are a type of accumulation that we definitely don't want to see in the body," says Kojima.

Basically, East Asian medicine focuses on the underlying causative factors. "We look at things like hot, cold, damp, dry in the environment affecting your body," says Ishii. "We would say external qi can affect the body and the organs, eventually impeding circulation and metabolism in a certain area. Maybe your qi is not strong enough to resolve that. Over time, that would cause pathological changes," says Ishii.

There's also an emotional side to this. Many cancer survivors report depression, anxiety, grief, and other emotional concerns, according to the Institute for Traditional Medicine. While Western medicine tends to treat these issues separately, East Asian medicine looks at physical and emotional concerns together.

East Asian medicine divides tumors into the types of patterns as they display. There are basically four types of masses in the East Asian vernacular:

- Phlegm masses
- Masses caused by heat accumulation
- Masses caused by cold accumulation
- Blood stasis masses

Typically, in the United States and other Western nations, a patient goes to Western health-care providers who diagnose and treat the cancer until they are in remission. At that point, they may turn to an East Asian practitioner, at least partly to recuperate from the Western treatment. "The Chinese doctor would say, you still have to go back and address the causative factor that led to the qi deficiency," says Ishii. "When they're finished with treatment, we help to address the causative factors that led to the masses."

Ishii also helps people handle the exhaustion and side effects associated with Western cancer treatments, helping patients maintain the strength to stick with the Western protocols. People usually come to Ishii, and other East Asian practitioners saying, "I'm just not the same person I used to be." They are typically exhausted, depressed, anxious, lacking much of an appetite, and complaining of generalized aches and pains, he says.

The Four Pillars

The four methods that East Asian medical practitioners use are as follows:

Acupuncture. This is the use of tools on the superficial aspect of the body to affect the flow of the qi in the body. "People think acupuncture is just needles," says Ishii. "But there are many tools for pressing. We have tools that press down on or tap the skin. Some of the ancient tools, which aren't used any longer, look more like surgical scalpels." I haven't experienced anything other than the basic needles, though.

The principle of manipulating the qi operates from the outside in, using gates of influence or acupoints along the meridians. "We stimulate the exterior of the body to affect the interior. This way, we can effect change along the path of the meridian or the related organ," says Ishii. "This is why we consider acupuncture a powerful form of orthopedic and internal medicine." By stimulating a specific meridian on the skin, acupuncturists can influence another spot, internal, along the pathway of qi circulation. This is how, says the Institute of for Traditional Medicine, inserting a needle in the hand can affect the intestines.

Acupuncturists study for years about how and where to insert the needles into precise spots, or pressure points. Acupuncture has been known to help cancer survivors with a wide range of symptoms, according to the National Center for Complementary and Alternative Medicine (NCCAM). These include:

- Joint pain and stiffness (especially for people taking aromatase inhibitors)
- Hot flashes (includes prostate and breast cancer survivors)
- Anxiety
- Depression
- Weight loss or gain
- Coughing and coughing up blood
- Speech problems
- Blocked esophagus
- Fluid in arms or legs[1]

---

1. "Acupuncture for Pain," *National Center for Complementary and Alternative Medicine*, last modified August 2010, http://nccam.nih.gov/health/acupuncture/acupuncture-for-pain.htm.

Acupuncture also includes a therapy called moxibustion, or moxa. When the dried herb, mugwort, is burned, the warmth stimulates circulation, and the smoke is believed to purge impurities out of the body, boost the immune system, and decrease pain. This is a strong form of treatment and can be used in several forms: "au naturale," purified into a fine powder, or made into a moxa stick, which looks kind of like a small cigar. Usually, at least in the United States, the acupuncturist burns it just above—not on—the body. Ishii uses moxa on me in two ways: resting a small cone on my stomach and then on the tip of acupuncture needles. Once the moxa is sitting there, he burns it, but, don't worry, it doesn't burn me; all I get is a little ash to flick aside. While it is burning, the moxa feels warm and soothing, with a smell sort of like pot, though a little less sweet. It fills the room with smoke, despite the air filter, which doesn't bother me, though it did make my eyes tear a little the first time. Somehow, having bits of mugwort burning just over my body is strangely soothing and relaxing. As I get up from the table, I have to flick a few ashes from my legs, not what I usually expect from a visit to a health-care provider. The aroma of the moxa stays with me for a while, even after I leave the office, and sometimes I get a few strange looks on the subway.

As proponents continue to spread the word, acupuncture has become more and more accepted in the United States. As of this writing, more than forty states and the District of Columbia have passed laws regulating acupuncture practice. Most require certification from the National Certification Commission for Acupuncture and Oriental Medicine.

As for moxa, the American Cancer Society has determined that it is safe, as long as you don't ingest it or have it burned directly on skin.[2] There are few research studies that look at moxa used in

---

2. "Moxibustion," *American Cancer Society*, last modified March 8, 2011, http://www.cancer.org/treatment/treatmentsandsideeffects/complementaryandalternativemedicine/manualhealingandphysicaltouch/moxibustion.

conjunction with acupuncture, so Western medicine can't "prove" its effectiveness, but if you try it and it helps you, that may be "proof" enough for you.

Nutrition and Herbal Therapy. "We actually see nutrition and herbal medicine on a continuum," says Kojima. They help strengthen the flow of qi in similar ways, she explains, but herbal medicine is much stronger. That's why you take herbs in small pill-sized doses, but eat food three times a day, at least. "You don't want to have too much of herbs," she says.

Traditional Chinese medicine emphasizes fresh, whole foods, rather than items that are synthetic, processed, or refined, according to the Pacific College of Oriental Medicine. Think about organic foods, seasonal fruits and vegetables, and fresh fish and meat. Also recommended are sprouted grains, beans, and vinegar (but not white vinegar, which is processed). "Try to have something pickled, or sauerkraut, every day," Ishii recommends.

TCM also emphasizes warm, cooked food that is easily digested. "If you must use your own qi to cook the food internally, this can weaken the digestion over time. For a sick patient who is already qi depleted, this is further debilitating," says Ishii. "When your qi is already depleted, it's better to avoid raw foods."

"We find it important to talk about things that shouldn't be eaten," says Kojima, "as well as things that should be eaten." In general, TCM recommends avoiding anything with partially hydrogenated oils, trans fatty acids, sugar, high fructose corn syrup, white flour, or refined carbohydrates. Skip the additives, coloring, or other artificial ingredients. This sounds very much like the AICR recommendations. In addition, TCM recommends avoiding

- Alcohol
- Processed foods
- Coffee (regular and decaffeinated)
- Cheese and other dairy

- Eggs
- Greasy, fatty, and oily foods
- Red meat
- Very spicy foods

Whole, organic foods in their simplest forms are seen as healing substances. They nourish your body, according to Pacific College, and help bring it into balance.[3] TCM also emphasizes the "seventy percent" rule. In other words, eat until you feel about seventy percent full. The idea is that this approach will compensate for the fact that it takes about twenty minutes for the brain to recognize a full stomach. If you give your brain a chance to catch up with your stomach, the theory goes, you can avoid unhealthy weight gain and maintain the body's energy balance. You might even lose a little weight.

Similarly, ingesting healing herbs helps bring the body into balance and gain qi. The qi then flows out through the blood stream to affect the body. Basically, this works in reverse of acupuncture—from the inside out. Some herbs are food items, but not all are, explains Ishii. Herbs can include twigs, branches, leaves, animal parts, and minerals. By the way, you don't end up with little baggies of mystery twigs and leaves; East Asian herbs often come in pill form—much easier to swallow, if less exotic looking.

This pillar of Eastern medicine is particularly important for cancer patients, because, even if your Western cancer docs aren't comfortable with herbal supplements, you still have to eat. "If you see food as a way to affect your metabolism," points out Ishii, "you could do it three times a day at least," without having to go to the gym, buy special equipment, or change your life in a major way.

---

3.   Alex A. Kecskes, "Eastern Nutrition and Whole Foods," *Pacific College of Oriental Medicine*, accessed December 4, 2013, http://www.pacificcollege.edu/acupuncture-massage-news/articles/440-eastern-nutrition-and-whole-foods.html.

According to the Institute for Traditional Medicine, these are some of the herbs most frequently prescribed to cancer survivors:

- Sophora Root. Believed to inhibit the growth of sarcoma-180, which in turn is believed to inhibit tumors.
- Oldenlandia. Used in removing toxins, especially used for cervical, breast, and rectal tumors.
- Curcuma and Zedoria. Believed to shrink tumors and often used for cervical cancer. Also helpful for promoting circulation during radiation treatment.
- Oyster Shell. Can soften and dissolve masses in the body.
- Astragalus. Believed to restore immune functions and attack cancer cells.
- Millettia. Used to restore red and white blood cell counts that have been depressed because of, say, chemotherapy.[4]

Herbal supplements garner the most concern of the four East Asian medical pillars among Western docs. According to the National Center for Complementary and Alternative Medicine (NCCAM), not all herbal treatments are safe—and some have been contaminated with toxins, heavy metals, or other ingredients not listed on the bottle.

NCCAM has also expressed concern that some herbs can interact with other medication and can have serious side effects. For instance, the center notes that the Chinese herb ephedra has been linked to heart attack and stroke; the ingredient has been banned by the FDA, though the ban does not apply to TCM remedies or herbal teas.[5] You should always let your oncology doctors know if you're taking herbs, and what you are taking, to be sure that they don't interfere with what they're prescribing.

---

4. Subhuti Dharmananda, "Oriental Perspectives on Cancer and Its Treatment," *Institute for Traditional Medicine*, May 1997, http://www.itmonline.org/arts/cancer.htm.

5. "Ephedra," *National Center for Complementary and Alternative Medicine*, last modified June 2013, http://nccam.nih.gov/health/ephedra.

Kojima recommends seeing an herbalist for a prescription that addresses your specific needs. At the same time, NCCAM suggests that you also discuss any herbal treatments with your onco docs. Herbs are a powerful form of Eastern medicine, so just check it out before you put any into your body.

Qigong. Translated as "qi practice," qigong uses mind and body to create more qi in a person, says Kojima. It includes breathing techniques, gentle movement, and meditation to cleanse, strengthen, and circulate the qi throughout the body. "Qigong is very useful because source qi is very hard to rejuvenate and qigong is the only way to do it," says Ishii.

Though a review of scientific studies indicates that qigong isn't proven to be effective in cancer care,[6] it might well improve quality of life. Research at The University of Texas MD Anderson Cancer Center found that qigong can reduce depressive symptoms and improves quality of life in women undergoing radiotherapy for breast cancer.

Qigong is relatively gentle, says Kojima. That's why people can offer classes in the practice for anyone who wants to come. "Classes usually involve general practices that promote overall qi," says Kojima.

There's also the notion of medical qigong, she explains, which is geared to the particular person. For instance, someone who has had lung cancer might be prescribed a qigong practice that focuses on breathing. "When you're prescribed a very specific qigong practice, you shouldn't necessarily go and have all your friends do it with you," she explains.

For example, if someone has heartburn or acid reflux, a practitioner might focus on moving the qi back down, rather than

---

6.   Lee et al., "Qigong for Cancer Treatment: A Systematic Review of Controlled Clinical Trials," *National Center for Biotechnology Information* 46 (2007): 717–22. www.ncbi.nlm.nih.gov/pubmed/17653892.

having it continue to flow up. Now, if someone else, say, with diarrhea, does this practice, it wouldn't work out so well. Someone with diarrhea is having no problem with qi moving downward; if anything, that person needs a little bit of upward shift in qi. So, says Kojima, using an inappropriate type of medical qigong could actually be harmful. In other words, as with Western medicine, don't share your prescriptions.

Physical Manipulation. This pillar, which is sometimes called Tui-Na, Thai massage, Thai yoga, or assisted yoga, is typically used less often than the others in treating cancer patients and survivors.

"The third pillar developed out of martial arts and also out of religious traditions," says Ishii. Basically, the goal is stretching and deep tissue massage. It also includes acupressure, hand massage, and partner-assisted stretches and directly affects the musculature. "Very honestly there is sometimes a joint adjustment that happens, but that's not necessarily what we're trying to do," says Ishii.

Massage allows East Asian practitioners to direct the qi in a specific way. "We can also release areas of congestion and tightening," says Kojima. Massage is particularly helpful in working with any tightening in the muscle areas. "Again, it's ultimately about wanting qi to be balanced and flowing regularly," says Kojima. This modality also includes liniments and plasters, administered externally. (If you swallow them, they're considered herbal therapy.)

Just like Western medicine, East Asian medicine is a medical system with several components that work well together or independently. Not every cancer survivor experiences the "joys" of radiation; similarly, not every patient of East Asian medicine experiences all the four "pillars" of the practice. In fact, there's a good chance that cancer patients will not be treated with physical manipulation. The key is, just as with Western medicine, to be guided by a skilled practitioner who knows just what will help you the most, and to let your oncology doctors know what you're up to, to be sure that it won't negatively affect your treatment or recuperation.

Frequently Asked Questions

Q: What is East Asian medicine? Is it one of those New Age, hippie things?

A: East Asian medicine is a longstanding system of health care designed to heal the body, mind, and spirit. Actually, it consists of a large number of systems, though TCM (traditional Chinese medicine) is the best-known variety in the United States.

Q: Does acupuncture hurt? Will I look like a porcupine?

A: Acupuncturists use a variety of instruments—mostly needles these days—to pinpoint precise spots on the body, called meridians. So there might be one needle in your wrist, and another near your ankle. And while you feel a quick prick when the needle goes in, it doesn't hurt after that.

Q: Are herbs safe to take with other medication?

A: In China and other East Asian countries, people use a combination of Western medicine and herbal treatments. But in the West, health-care providers aren't as knowledgeable about Eastern modalities. The safest bet is to speak with your Western cancer docs before starting with any Eastern herbal remedies.

Q: What is qigong? Does it have to be one-on-one? I've seen classes offered.

A: Qigong combines breathing, movement, and meditation. If you work with someone one-on-one, you'll receive more individualized attention than if you take a class, but both are beneficial.

Q: What is qi? Or is it chi?

A: The term is usually written "qi" and pronounced "chee." People often translate it as "energy," but it is much more. Eastern medicine sees qi as life force, the thing that maintains your equilibrium.

Chapter 15

Other Complementary Approaches

Beth (not me), a New York City property manager, has always internalized her stress. She'd done so even before cancer entered her life. But once it did, she had even more stress to internalize. After nine years of surgical biopsies that turned out to be nothing, she was "finally" diagnosed with breast cancer on the left side; she was treated with a lumpectomy and radiation. The following year, the cancer recurred on the right side . . . another lumpectomy. Then the next year, the doctors found cancer, again, on her left side.

At this point, her doctors recommended mastectomy. "I freaked out, of course," Beth says. "I freaked out because I was really attached to my boobs, and I didn't want to give them up. I've had relatively big boobs all my life, and it was so much a part of my identity and my self-esteem," she adds.

She ended up with a bilateral mastectomy and reconstruction. It required a huge fight with her insurance company, which, of course, only added to the tension level. The good news was that her chances of having any more breast cancer were pretty small. The bad news: she was stressed.

Beth wasn't sure what to do about it. She turned to some complementary modalities, notably massage, acupuncture, reflexology, and aromatherapy. She enrolled in a program at You Can Thrive, a non-profit organization which, at that time, offered a three-month free program for breast cancer survivors.

Complementary modalities, also called CAM and integrated medicine, is basically a catch-all term for a variety of health-care approaches developed outside of Western medicine. Beth was predisposed to be comfortable with these types of treatments. "Even before the surgery, I sort of leaned toward massage and reflexology," says Beth.

But they became more powerful tools when her need for them increased. "They help you find how to balance your life and center yourself," she explains. "Because if you're so stressed and you're not sleeping and you're not eating, your whole body's out of whack."

"The first day I was there, I walked out of the You Can Thrive office feeling like I was stoned," says Beth. "Because I was, all of a sudden, so relaxed." She found that the weekly sessions were very useful. "It just helped you to have time to focus on something else or to clear your mind, really," says Beth. "It was almost like a meditation."

Uses of Complementary Modalities

Beth is not the only one who feels this way. The Centers for Disease Control and Prevention (CDC) found that about two out of every three cancer survivors turned to a complementary approach, usually for general wellness, immune enhancement, or pain management.[1] When

---

1. Nahin et al., "Costs of Complementary and Alternative Medicine (CAM) and Frequency of Visits to CAM Practitioners: United States, 2007," *Centers for Disease Control and Prevention* (2009): 18. www.cdc.gov/nchs/data/nhsr/nhsr018.pdf.

a survivor combines Western medicine with complementary therapy, it is called integrative medicine—sort of the best of both worlds.

People have found that complementary approaches are particularly helpful for alleviating the long-term effects of cancer and its treatment—quality of life issues such as fatigue, anxiety, and depression. There is less research, unfortunately, indicating that it lowers the risk of cancer.

When we say "complementary approaches," we're talking about a wide range of modalities. Many of them are centuries old. Think, for instance, about yoga, acupuncture, herbs, and massage. The National Center for Complementary and Alternative Medicine (NCCAM), which is part of the National Institutes of Health (NIH), divides complementary modalities into three types:

- Natural products (such as vitamin supplements and probiotics)
- Mind and body medicine (including meditation, guided imagery, and journaling)
- Manipulative and body-based practices (think about massage therapy, reiki, and yoga)[2]

I'd like to add a fourth category for this chapter: psychosocial support, which, I suggest, includes support groups and individual therapy.

CAM modalities are most helpful, experts say, when used in conjunction with Western medicine. It is always best, though, to talk with your health-care provider to make sure there are no potentially problematic consequences from these non-Western approaches you might want to explore.

Specifically, some complementary health approaches can interfere with Western medicine; for instance, according to NCCAM, the herb

---

2. "Complementary, Alternative, or Integrative Health: What's In a Name?" *National Center for Complementary and Alternative Medicine*, last modified May 2013, http://nccam.nih.gov/health/whatiscam.

St. John's wort can render some Western medicines less effective.[3] Perhaps more concerning is that some complementary modalities can actually cause harm; the NCCAM points to the example of massaging an area that was directly affected by radiation. Ouch. That's one more reason to go to a credentialed, skilled practitioner.

Natural Products

Vitamin Supplements

A large number of cancer survivors take vitamin supplements. I was told to take calcium supplements, for instance.

Overall, there are thirteen vitamins (A, C, D, E, K, and B vitamins) and a bunch of minerals (notably calcium, phosphorus, magnesium, iron, zinc, and selenium) that human beings need to be healthy. When these vitamins and minerals come in pill or tablet form, as opposed to broccoli or carrots, they're called supplements.

Vitamin supplementation can be a controversial topic. According to the National Center for Complementary and Alternative Medicine (NCCAM) as well as the American Institute for Cancer Research (AICR), some doctors are concerned about cancer survivors taking supplements. They recommend sticking with food, and emphasizing fruits and vegetables (see Chapter 13: Nutrition). The institute points out that some studies have found that supplements can upset the balance of nutrients in the body.[4]

That doesn't mean that all supplements are bad, says Alice Bender, MS, RD, nutrition communications manager at AICR. "People over age fifty may need B-12; people living in northern climates may need vitamin D; the elderly may need calcium," she adds. "But in general,

---

3. "St. John's Wort and Depression," *National Center for Complementary and Alternative Medicine,* last modified September 2012, http://nccam.nih.gov/health/stjohnswort/sjw-and-depression.htm?

4. "Phytochemicals: The Cancer Fighters in the Foods We Eat," *American Institute for Cancer Research,* April 10, 2013, http://www.aicr.org/reduce-your-cancer-risk/diet/elements_phytochemicals.html

the American Institute for Cancer Research feels that the overall diet is more important than the individual components in preventing cancer."

Probiotics

Called beneficial bacteria or "friendly germs," probiotics are live micro-organisms intended to maintain the health of your intestinal track and aid in digestion. The idea is that they keep potentially harmful bacteria and yeasts under control. Basically, they take over the small intestine and crowd out the bad stuff. I've been taking them for a while, though, honestly, I haven't noticed any changes as a result.

Probiotics are thought to

- Aid acute diarrhea and antibiotic-associated diarrhea
- Improve atopic eczema
- Boost immunity

Most probiotics come from food sources, especially cultured milk products, according to the Susan G. Komen Foundation.[5] There are a wide range of probiotic bacteria, and different probiotics can have varying effects on different people. They usually come in caplets and tablet form, though you can also find them in beverages, powders, yogurt, and many fermented foods, such as sauerkraut and kimchi.

The U.S. Food and Drug Administration (FDA), which regulates food and medications, does not oversee supplements such as probiotics, so there's no guarantee about any variety's purity, safety, or strength.[6] Experts recommend talking with your oncology docs about taking probiotics to be sure they don't interact with any of the medications you are taking.

---

5. "Probiotics," *Susan G. Komen Foundation*, accessed December 4, 2013, http://ww5.komen.org/BreastCancer/Probiotics.html.

6. "Dietary Supplements," *Food and Drug Administration*, last modified August 28, 2013, http://www.fda.gov/food/dietarysupplements/.

Mind and Body Medicine

Meditation

After I finished treatment for Hodgkin's disease, I took a class in mindfulness-based stress reduction (MBSR), a style of meditation developed by John Kabat-Zinn, PhD, at the University of Massachusetts Medical Center specifically to help people deal with chronic illness or pain. For ten weeks, I practiced focusing my attention, intently, on the moment. Our teacher led us through meditation exercises, gentle stretches, and small-group conversation.

I'm not sure I ever fully "got" the techniques. Ten weeks is probably not enough time. When trying them on the subway, I meditated just as much on the order of the stops and whether I'd missed my station as I did on being mindful of the moment. In class, I had a very hard time concentrating for five full minutes on a raisin in my hand.

But I do believe that the process of trying, albeit trying and failing, was useful. With my mind fighting off the effects of chemobrain, it helped to focus only on one thing. The process of talking about how to focus, and how to forgive ourselves for not doing it perfectly, gave me a regular respite from thinking about cancer. Thinking about thinking is quite a different phenomenon, and one that is much less anxiety-provoking. "It's about paying attention on purpose to what we want to pay attention to," says Elaine Retholz, certified MBSR instructor—currently the only one teaching in New York City.

The practice emphasizes showing compassion toward yourself and others. The goal, and Retholz emphasizes that it is an ever-evolving practice, is to "begin to cultivate paying attention with kindness and curiosity and interest."

The benefits of MBSR, reportedly, are

- Increased ability to cope with short- and long-term stress
- Increased ability to relax

- Decreases in pain levels
- Enhanced ability to cope with chronic pain
- Greater energy and enthusiasm[7]

One thing we humans do well is focusing on pain. "We touch our tooth to see if it still hurts," says Retholz. MBSR allows practitioners to put their attention where they want it to be. But that's not to suggest that MBSR should replace dentistry, only that if you can't get an appointment until next Tuesday, MBSR might help you hang on until then.

The same meditation approach works for fear of recurrence. "Mindfulness is about being in the present moment, to focus on what's happening now, and we don't have to imagine what might happen in the future," says Retholz. Again, MBSR is not a replacement for standard oncology treatment and follow-up. It's just a tool for getting through it and coping with survivorship.

In the class I took, we focused our attention during the session and in homework assignments. But the goal is not strictly to be able to meditate for twenty minutes a day. The idea is to hone a skill that you can whip out of your tool box as needed.

Retholz likens meditation practice to practicing the piano. "You repeat the scales over and over and over again. It's not so that you get really good at scales; it's so that you can play music," she says. "That way, in difficult circumstances, we don't have to spin out; we can be present in the same way," she explains. The idea is to develop a certain mental agility. "We're training our minds."

Guided Imagery

"Close your eyes. Sit comfortably and don't cross your arms or legs. Feel your breath as it comes in and out, in and out. Try to relax and picture a safe place. . . ."

---

7. "What is Mindfulness-Based Stress Reduction?" *Mindful Living Programs*, accessed December 5, 2013, http://www.mindfullivingprograms.com/whatMBSR.php.

That is how some guided imagery sessions begin, though there are countless approaches. Guided imagery, also called visualization, is a technique used by a therapist in a group or one-on-one. Sessions usually last twenty to thirty minutes. Like meditation, guided imagery can help increase self-awareness and focus your mind.

Typically, the therapist will guide you to envision places or situations that help you feel safe and secure, or perhaps think about a spirit guide. The therapist may describe the sounds, smells, tastes, or other sensations that are part of the scene. Often, you are asked to focus on your body in the moment. There may be gentle background music. It can be soothing and can give you a chance to really focus on thinking through issues without getting side tracked by daily life.

Some studies, according to the American Cancer Society, have shown that guided imagery can help

- Deal with stress
- Decrease anxiety
- Improve depression
- Lower blood pressure
- Reduce pain[8]

Reiki

"I've seen people have all kinds of responses—deep emotional responses, physical responses," says Annalise Evanson, MA, MBA, ARCB, CPCC, CPWC. Evanson is a holistic energy practitioner and teacher who holds certifications in Usui and Karuna Reiki.

"It seems to be a modality that, from an energetic perspective, what I call a vibrational perspective, seems to reach people where they're at and help something shift, move," she says. "It gives you what you need right then and there."

---

8. "Imagery," *American Cancer Society*, last modified November 1, 2008, http://www.cancer.org/treatment/treatmentsandsideeffects/complementaryandalterna-tivemedicine/mindbodyandspirit/imagery.

A Japanese technique, Reiki gently helps restore wellness and balance to survivors on physical, emotional, mental, and spiritual levels. It is meant to reduce stress and promote relaxation and healing. A practitioner uses her hands to transfer energy to the survivor. There are several styles of Reiki, and many practitioners use a combination of two or more. A typical session lasts about an hour.

Reiki works by directing the flow of life force in order to move negative psychic energy out of the body and channel healing energies, according to the International Center for Reiki Training. "It is intuitive," says Evanson. "It's like a laying on of hands."

Practitioners use about a dozen different hand positions, holding their hands one or two inches above the clothed survivor. They hold each position for two to five minutes. Sessions can focus on treating a specific concern or promoting overall well-being.

It is thought that Reiki can do the following:

- Relieve pain
- Decrease depression and anxiety
- Promote relaxation and a sense of well-being[9]

There hasn't been any scientific research on the effectiveness of Reiki. It is considered safe, says the American Cancer Society, with no worrisome risks or side effects.

Journaling

Writing down your innermost thoughts and feelings can help you express those emotions that are, sometimes, too painful to say out loud, especially to an audience. It can help you find ways to gain some control over your life, and to think through your relationships. It can be a very helpful approach for sorting out your feelings, thinking through problems, and becoming more hopeful about the future.

9. "Reiki," *American Cancer Society*, last modified March 8, 2012, http://www.cancer .org/treatment/treatmentsandsideeffects/complementaryandalternativemedicine/ manualhealingandphysicaltouch/reiki.

"Some people might need to write in their journals because they're not able to process very easily by talking but instead need to think about it in their own heads, and maybe write it down," says Hannah H. Gibson-Moore, LMSW, emotional support counselor at the Livestrong Foundation.

There's no "right" way to journal. You can do it every day, every week, or every month—whatever feels right. You can focus on day-to-day activities or on your emotions. You can use it to look for the positive, or to complain about the negative. You can take the traditional paper-and-pencil approach or type on a computer; don't forget to put a password on your journal, though, if you want privacy. And you can keep a journal for yourself only, or to communicate with others.

There are several different types of journaling, not limited to the following:

- **Stream-of-Consciousness Writing.** This approach is raw. You just write down your thoughts and emotions, without a thought to grammar or structure. No editing is allowed.
- **Art Journaling.** This is more like a scrapbook of sketching, drawing, or doodling. Anything goes if it helps you feel as though you've gotten your thoughts out of your brain and onto paper.
- **Gratitude Journaling.** This type of journal contains only positive entries and affirmations. Some people find this a way to focus their minds on the positive.

Some people also keep a daily, weekly, or periodic blog to communicate their thoughts and feelings with others. The catch is that while you can get away with the occasional typo, if your goal is communication, you will need to express yourself clearly. Blogs can be short snippets of thoughts or longer pieces, whatever is most helpful to you.

Often, it is helpful to write in a quiet space where you know you will have at least fifteen to twenty minutes of uninterrupted time. You might want to keep it someplace private, so that you know your thoughts and emotions will be safe from prying eyes. Don't edit yourself; who cares about grammar, spelling, or sentence structure? No one else is going to read this, right? The key is to remember that you are keeping a journal for yourself. It doesn't have to be of any use to anyone else.

Some research has shown that keeping a daily journal can have positive effects on your health and quality of life. A recent study also shows that bloggers who "chronicle their experience and communicate with their social network via the Internet," also benefit.[10] In fact, in a blog entry, Kathy-Ellen Kups, RN, writes, "I definitely find that sharing openly on the web helps keep me sane about my thoughts on the disease."

Manipulative and Body-Based Practices

Massage

Beth (not me) found that massage "really helped" her deal with the pain and anxiety of survivorship. It was soothing and relaxing, and took her mind off the emotional and logistical challenges of life after cancer, at least temporarily. It worked this way for me, too, while I was going through chemotherapy. It's not surprising, as massage is one of the most popular complementary approaches. The modality is centuries old and involves the manipulation of soft tissue.

With massage, practitioners use their hands, and sometimes forearms, elbows, and massage tools, to manipulate soft tissue. Most sessions last thirty to sixty minutes, and practitioners often dim the lights and pipe in soothing music to set a relaxing mood.

---

10. Stanton et al., "Project Connect Online: Randomized Trial of an Internet-Based Program to Chronicle the Cancer Experience and Facilitate Communication," *National Center for Biotechnology Information* (2013): 3411–7. doi: 10.1200/JCO.2012.46.9015.

Massage comes in a variety of flavors, including Swedish massage, sports massage, neuromuscular therapy, and myotherapy. Swedish massage is probably the most common style used in the United States, though most massage therapists combine several styles and techniques.

According to NCCAM, massage can decrease:

- Stress
- Anxiety
- Depression
- Pain
- Fatigue[11]

Not only that—the National Cancer Institute has found that massage can also

- Release endorphins, which relieve pain and provide a sense of well-being
- Increase the flow of blood and lymphatic fluid
- Improve the effectiveness of pain medications
- Decrease inflammation and edema[12]

Massage is generally considered safe, says the American Cancer Society. Therapists should be gentle with bones that have been weakened by metastasis, and with patients with low platelet counts, as there could be bruising, and be cautious with skin damaged by radiation. Also, if you've had breast reconstruction and have been told not to lie on your stomach, be aware that there's no exception

---

11. "Massage Therapy," *National Center for Complementary and Alternative Medicine*, last modified August 2010, http://nccam.nih.gov/health/massage/massageintroduction.htm.

12. "Massage," *American Cancer Society*, last modified May 23, 2013, http://www.cancer.org/treatment/treatmentsandsideeffects/complementaryandalternative-medicine/manualhealingandphysicaltouch/massage.

to this rule for massage. Just check with your cancer docs, but in general, massage is safe and soothing. Some hospitals offer it routinely to cancer patients and survivors.

Yoga

Khit ran away from home when she was sixteen years old to avoid an arranged marriage to her first cousin, orchestrated by her "old-school Palestinian" parents. She made it through high school by working two or three jobs at a time. "I lived in my car and on people's couches when times got rough," she says. She had a couple of relationships that were verbally and physically abusive, and then at age twenty-six, she was diagnosed with vulval cancer. But she was so busy earning a living, getting through high school, and regaining her health that she never really had the chance to deal with her difficult history.

A friend took her to yoga class one time, but it wasn't her thing. "I hated it. I said, 'I can't do this, I'm not sweating, I'm not burning calories, this is a waste of my fricking time.' I hated it," she says.

But then she was diagnosed with melanoma, her second primary cancer. Her boyfriend at the time—who knew she was already a cancer survivor—stood her up at the hospital. "He finally told me that he realized that his job was more important to him than to be there for me for cancer," she says. "He said he knew he wasn't going to be that person for me, so he broke up with me."

Khit felt suicidal. She held onto a bottle of Xanax and considered whether perhaps that was the way to go. "I didn't want to go through any more pain," she remembers. "I just wanted someone to come home to. I wanted someone I could put down as an emergency contact on whatever form I was filling out," Khit says. She sat in her apartment for days and days and didn't talk to anyone. Her grades suffered, and she didn't show up for her jobs. She realized she had to do something. "I didn't want medicine, and I didn't want to go to a therapist." So she figured she'd give yoga a try again.

This time, she had a different teacher, and a completely different experience.

"Yoga was the first thing that allowed me to start breathing and really sit back and think a lot about what happened to me," she says. "When I'm in yoga, I can calm down and breathe. There are no cell phones, no distractions. So I'm forced to deal with my own thoughts," she says. Her teacher talks about appreciation and gratitude.

"Because of her and because of yoga, I have been able to transform myself," says Khit. "This time last year, I was trying to make sense of why I was alive." Her entire attitude has changed. "Now I see that I am the captain of my own ship. And I can choose who I want on my boat," says Khit.

An ancient Hindu practice, dating back more than five thousand years, yoga combines exercises, controlled breathing, and meditation. It is designed to strengthen both mind and body. Practitioners take poses that can be physically challenging (in my opinion, this includes anything where you have to hold your feet above your head) or very relaxing (such as child's pose or downward facing dog).

There are more than one hundred different types of yoga practiced in the United States, according to the American Cancer Society. Hatha yoga, though, is most popular for cancer survivors because it has relatively easy movements and a relaxed pace. There are even classes in sitting yoga, intended for survivors with low flexibility and energy.

Studies, notes the American Cancer Society, have shown that yoga can:

- Decrease blood pressure
- Decrease heart rate
- Improve energy levels and manage fatigue
- Improve mood
- Decrease stress levels

- Increase muscle strength
- Improve flexibility
- Aid in balance
- Lower depression and anxiety
- Decrease stress[13]

The American Cancer Society warns that survivors who are dehydrated could run into trouble with Bikram yoga, which is an energetic style of yoga typically practiced in a hot room, often about 100 degrees Fahrenheit. But other than that, NCCAM finds yoga to be safe when practiced appropriately.

Reflexology

"Reflexology is based on the theory that your entire body is mirrored on your hands, on your feet, and in your ears," says Annalise Evanson, who is nationally board certified in reflexology, as teacher and practitioner, in addition to her Reiki practice. "The theory behind the work is that when you're working on the hands or feet or ears, even though it feels good because you're working on tissue, you're actually working on the map of the body," she explains. The feet, for instance, contain 7,200 nerves, twenty-six bones, and thirty-three joints, she notes. And who doesn't like having their feet rubbed?

Reflexology is a non-invasive practice involving thumb and finger techniques to apply alternating pressure to reflexes shown on reflex maps of the body located on the feet, hands, and outer ears. Practitioners don't use any tools, though sometimes they apply lotion. The average session lasts about an hour.

Evanson explains that reflexology

- Promotes relaxation
- Reduces stress

---

13. "Yoga," *American Cancer Society*, last modified November 1, 2008, http://www .cancer.org/treatment/treatmentsandsideeffects/complementaryandalternative medicine/mindbodyandspirit/yoga.

- Promotes circulation
- Helps with pain

Psychosocial Support

Support Groups

I joined a support group by accident. With my Hodgkin's diagnosis coming three months on the heels of a difficult marital separation, my daughter—then ten years old—was angry. Really angry. I didn't know what to do.

Audrey, a friend and breast cancer survivor whose son was in my son's class at the time, told me, "The one thing I regret about when I was going through treatment is that we didn't go to Gilda's Club." Gilda's offers a variety of services for people touched by cancer, but one of the major activities is support groups for survivors, children, and caregivers.

I was and remain in awe of Audrey. She's brilliant and funny, highly professional, and very compassionate. If she thought Gilda's was a good thing, I had to check it out. I applied and signed all three of us up. I told my children, "I have to do something about the cancer upstairs and while I'm up there, you can play with the kids downstairs."

I admit it—I lied. It was actually the other way around. I joined for the kids and then, because I didn't want it to be a *total* lie, I joined the adult group. I didn't need it—of course—I was coping just fine, I told myself. I just went for the kids.

Later, I 'fessed up and (thank goodness) was forgiven.

Anyway, all three of us went a little reluctantly the first week. My son, Ari, then six years old, loved it from day one—a room full of games, kids, and adults ready to play. Sometimes there was a visitor—a cartoonist, specially trained dogs—and sometimes there was a special building or art project. But always there were snacks. (No fair; they didn't feed the adults upstairs.) One of the volunteers,

Natasha, made a killer chocolate birthday cake. Noogieland, as it is called, was a big hit with my son.

My daughter Maya, though, sat in a corner, shielded by her scooter, and read for two hours, for the first few sessions.

Fortunately, Ari acted as ambassador. He pulled Maya in, first for snack time, then to join him in a game because no one else would play Connect Four with him. You see, he always won, and while I took that as a challenge—I was convinced I'd eventually beat my first-grader—I could appreciate that the kids found his skill level frustrating. Eventually, Maya became involved with the other kids and made some friends that she saw outside of the group. For them, cancer became "normalized"; they weren't the only ones touched by the "C" word, and, in fact, they were some of the lucky ones. I was alive and going to remain so.

Meanwhile, upstairs, I was learning that a support group, especially led by a highly skilled facilitator, is really helpful. A group of mostly women, all in or just finished with treatment, we sat around in comfy chairs and sofas and talked. Sometimes we did updates, going around the circle; sometimes we just chatted more informally.

I gained some practical suggestions about foods to try when I was feeling particularly chemo nauseated and a sense of what was going to be coming along next. Perhaps the best part, though, was the sense of camaraderie. I wasn't going it alone anymore. Some of the members are still friends to this day, outside of the group, six years later.

In mid-November, we went around the circle talking about our plans for Thanksgiving. The kids and I didn't have any. We had no invitations, and I wasn't a great cook even before chemotherapy messed with my taste buds. Plus I was exhausted. I'd just finished with treatment and was feeling thankful for that, but not having holiday plans made me feel alone.

Another woman in the support group, who loved to cook and who had a daughter downstairs in Noogieland, was also upset. She had planned to celebrate finishing treatment by having her father come to Thanksgiving dinner, making it a real family celebration. But he had just cancelled because of work obligations.

She looked at me, I looked at her, and she invited the children and me to join her, family's Thanksgiving dinner. It sounded perfect; I really liked her, and our children got along well downstairs.

I started to cry. Then she started to cry. We'd both just finished treatment, and were feeling grateful for our survival and our families. I was appreciative to be invited to a lovely family event—and probably the yummiest Thanksgiving dinner I've ever had. It was certainly the one that inspired the most gratitude.

Eventually, my kids were ready to move on from Gilda's. They'd come to terms with my cancer diagnosis and treatment, I was healthy, and, more to the point, they were older and had other things to do with their Wednesday nights. Even after we left, though, we went back to the Halloween festivities for a few years. Games, candy, and circus performers: who could say no?

I ended up joining another group—this one focused on survivorship, with some other Gilda grads. Yup, I really didn't need a support group. Wasn't useful at all.

I was really lucky, though. Not all support groups are created equal. Some are organized by types of cancer, some by gender, and some by stage of life, such as young patients' groups. Some, like Noogieland, focused on children of survivors or children who lost a parent. Other groups are geared toward caregivers. Some offer ongoing education. The group I'm in now focuses on survivorship and often has speakers come to talk about acupuncture, breathing, career issues, sexuality, laughing yoga, and other topics.

One woman I met had started out in a hospital-based support group that sort of backfired; it made her more sad and vulnerable. She didn't give up, though; she came to our group, which proved warm, welcoming, and helpful in terms of information and support. She was glad she hadn't just given up on the idea of support groups.

According to the American Cancer Society, support groups provide information, comfort, and coping skills. They reduce anxiety and offer a place to share common concerns. Some research, says the ACS, shows that support groups can reduce tension, anxiety, fatigue, and enhance the quality of life.[14] However, I've heard from other people that some groups are just depressing. It depends on the group and the facilitator. I was lucky; I got Laura! Also, some support groups geared toward heterosexuals may not meet the needs of gay or lesbian survivors.

Some groups happen by phone, and others operate online. While these approaches can be convenient, especially at certain points in treatment when you're feeling particularly tired, they also have their shortcomings. When chat rooms don't have facilitators, they can serve more as kvetch-a-thons than as supportive environments, says Lillie Shockney, RN, BS, MAS, professor and administrative director, Johns Hopkins Cancer Survivorship Programs. Sometimes people generalize from their own experiences to a different set of circumstances—and end up providing other survivors with incorrect information.

The American Cancer Society concurs with these concerns. Its website notes that "online support groups should be used with caution. This venue cannot always assure privacy or confidentiality, and the people involved may have no special training or qualifications, especially if the group takes place in an unmonitored chat room."[15]

It's not too hard to find a support group, though it can take some trial and error to find one that meets your needs. Many hospitals offer groups; Gilda's Club, the Livestrong Foundation, and CancerCare

---

14. "Support Groups," *American Cancer Society*, last modified January 16, 2013, http://www.cancer.org/treatment/treatmentsandsideeffects/complementaryan-dalternativemedicine/mindbodyandspirit/support-groups-cam.

15. Ibid.

have groups in multiple locations. Malecare offers support groups specifically for males, while Young Survival Coalition and Stupid Cancer focus on young adults. (See Appendix 1: Resources for Survivorship for more information and suggestions.) Remember, if a group doesn't provide you with support, regardless of how your best friend sees it, it's time to move on. The right group is out there, just waiting for you. You just have to find it.

Individual Therapy

For years, I've been lucky enough to enjoy one-on-one therapy. It has enabled me to sort out exactly what is bothering me about particular situations, what I can do about it, and what I (sometimes) just need to accept. I get practical suggestions from someone who's not as emotional involved and can help with (hopefully minor) attitude adjustments. Most commonly, it's a matter of having someone I respect saying to me, "Let it go."

Probably the best part, though, is knowing that for fifty minutes a week I get to take center stage. I can kvetch, joke, brag, and analyze— or a little of all three. Plus, I know that someone is listening. (Except for one short-lived experience when I was sure the guy deliberately forgot his hearing aid when I showed up at the door.) I was lucky to be seeing a therapist with a very practical and supportive approach as I tried to pull my life together after treatment. She also offered a bit of cheerleading, periodically, which was also greatly appreciated.

I've never had the chance to relax on a black leather couch, though. Usually, in my experience, you spend forty-five to fifty minutes chatting, usually sitting in a chair in the therapist's office. Therapists are mental health professionals, such as psychologists, psychiatrists, social workers, counselors, and marriage and family therapists. Some have a degree in psychology, counseling, or social work, and, hopefully, they have a lot of experience helping people. Just like with support groups, it's important to find someone you feel comfortable with; you don't buy the first dress on the rack, so why would you go with the first therapist you find?

Some therapists are psycho-oncologists. According to the American Psychosocial Oncology Society (APOS), "Psychosocial oncology is a distinct professional discipline that is evidence based, rooted in the science of caring and integral to quality cancer care."[16] Not every cancer survivor wants a therapist with a specifically oncological focus, but others find onco-psychologists to be invaluable.

"It really totally depends on the person," says Mindy Greenstein, who is, herself, a psycho-oncologist. "If you're somebody who feels like he really, really wants to talk with somebody who's had a lot of cancer experience, then you should go with that." It's interesting, though, that there's no specialty of therapists with training in heart disease or diabetes. As we've seen before, there's just something a little different about cancer.

Beyond traditional client-centered therapy, there are a few other options:

- Behavior modification therapy, which tries to replace problematic patterns of behavior patterns with healthier options.
- Cognitive therapy, which helps survivors change their "gremlins" or harmful internal messages and replace them with positive self-talk.
- Couples therapy, which involves both members of a marriage or partnership.
- Group therapy, which involves a bunch of people meeting regularly and led, as other types of therapy, by a trained mental health professional.

It's not just my personal experience. Research has shown that psychotherapy can enable a survivor to

---

16. "APOS Membership Code of Ethics," *American Psychosocial Oncology Society*, accessed December 4, 2013, http://www.apos-society.org/about/membership/APOS.Member.CodeofEthics.pdf

- Develop coping skills
- Improve quality of life
- Reduce anxiety
- Decrease depression[17]

While it's possible that psychotherapy can bring up painful issues, the whole point of it is to help survivors (and others) come to terms with them. I'm not sure that's a "downside" to therapy, other than cost. (If you look around, though, you can probably find some sliding-scale options, particularly with social workers.) Really, for me, it's always been like having a trained friend who is sympathetic yet analytic—and always in a way that is compassionate.

The many complementary medicine options available could be compared to a huge buffet. It's a vast selection at first, and you don't know where to start. When you walk around a little, you start to see the pattern: salads to the left, side dishes over here, baked potato fixings on the right. Then you start to weed out what you don't want and narrow down what you do. You can come back for dessert, for instance. Then you might take a little bit of many things to see what you like, then come back for more of what's really yummy. Alternately, you might see exactly what you want immediately and go help yourself to it. Either way, you figure out what suits your needs at the moment and chow down—without having to worry about calorie intake.

Think of these complementary approaches in the same way. It's a matter of instinct, followed by trial and error. "There are so many things out there, and it's about discovering or maybe exploring what's going to support you. Because, you know, there's no one size fits all," says Evanson.

---

17. "Psychotherapy," *American Cancer Society*, last modified November 1, 2008, http://www.cancer.org/treatment/treatmentsandsideeffects/complementaryandalterna-tivemedicine/mindbodyandspirit/psychotherapy.

You may realize that guided imagery isn't for you, for instance, or it could be exactly what you need to help you relax and focus on your life. If it works, you're set; if not, feel free to move on. One of the joys of life, after cancer is the opportunity it gives you to regain control over your life, and part of that is the ability to choose how you will heal and move forward in life.

Frequently Asked Questions

Q: I am overwhelmed. There are so many options—how do I pick what will work best for me?

A: There are lots of ways you can help yourself deal with the challenges of survivorship. It can be a little overwhelming at first, but just read about the different options, talk to people who've tried them, and see what sounds fun or comforting to you. If you try one option and find it isn't for you, there are plenty of other options out there!

Q: Can I do more than one thing?

A: Try as many modalities as you have time and energy for. You may find that certain approaches work at some points and not others. For instance, if you're in a support group of people finishing up treatment, you may find that you are ready to move on after you're a year or so out from treatment. Stick with what feels helpful and meaningful to you, where you are right now.

Q: I feel like I've lost control of my life during cancer treatment. How can I get it back?

A: Whether you like to write or talk, are public or private, are active or sedentary, there's an approach here to help you focus on yourself and regain your strength and sense of control. Take a look at these options—and others. It's an all-you-can-eat buffet.

Q: Should I tell my oncologist, radiation oncologist, or surgeon about using any of these approaches?

A: Experts recommend telling your doctors about any supplements, including probiotics, that you want to take to make sure they won't react badly with what your doctors are prescribing.

Afterword

Silver Linings, or Consolation Prizes

It was a week after my double mastectomy and reconstruction surgery, three days after I got home from the hospital, and I put on a pair of silver earrings and a black skirt, and stuffed my new breasts-formerly-known-as-thighs into a black eyelet blouse. I had to tilt my head down to put my earrings in, as I couldn't raise my arms, but I was determined.

Charlotte, my friend and Jewish mother stand-in for the evening, came right on time, and I buzzed her up to the apartment. After a brief chat, we headed back down the two flights of stairs to the street. Charlotte tried to help me down the stairs, but when she realized I wasn't going to let her, she went first, to break my fall should I stumble. I wasn't sure whether to be insulted by her lack of faith or touched by her concern. I have to admit, though, I was a little woozy, and the evening had just started. We hailed a taxi and headed down to the theater district.

I'd known about it for a few weeks by this point, but was still stunned. A fundraiser? For me? What were they thinking?

Fundraisers are for worthwhile causes, important people, and political candidates. I refuse to comment on whether there are overlaps across these groups. But, anyway, fundraisers aren't for people like me—single mom, small-time freelance writer, and three-time cancer survivor.

It's a good thing I wasn't in charge of planning the event, or encouraging people to attend.

Apparently my friends Mitria, Wendy, and Susan were sitting around worrying about me over a bowl of pasta with vodka sauce, trying to figure out how to help. We'd been in a cancer support group together for a few years. Ironically, I had thought I was ready to "graduate" from the group; I'd been cancer-free for long enough. I didn't need the support anymore and thought that perhaps they should use my space for someone else who needed it more.

They hit on the idea of holding a fundraiser for me, but then weren't quite sure how to do it. "Well, we could hold a donut sale," Susan apparently said, "or I could do my show."

By day, Susan is a teacher in the New York City Public Schools working with homebound kids, but after hours, she's a playwright and actor, with the latest production being her one-woman show, *Teacher in the House*. The hour-long production, which I'd seen before, talks about Susan's experience teaching special needs children, entwined with her own experiences with breast cancer. It's a lovely combination of laugh-out-loud funny and truly poignant stories, beautifully written, directed, and acted.

While I still couldn't understand why I warranted a fundraiser, it did make perfect sense to me that a fundraiser held in New York City would involve a theatrical performance. And, better yet, an amazing one.

My friends found a small, forty-seat venue, spread the word, arranged for online ticket sales (which I have been told sold out hours before the performance!), and operated a small concessions stand before the show started. A friend, Deni, somehow found some extra folding chairs to squeeze in a few more bodies. Another friend, Roberta, got my synagogue involved, too. I was utterly astounded, thrilled, honored, and perplexed at this amazing outpouring of generosity. (I say this fully aware of the risk of sounding like a walking thesaurus.)

I was touched beyond words—which amused Mitria no end. "Beth, the writer, had nothing to say," she joked, as I struggled to hold back tears, not for the first—nor the last—time that evening. The show was wonderful as always (I wobbled to my feet to give a standing ovation), the audience enthusiastic and supportive (so many kind and gentle hugs), but probably the biggest gift was knowing that I am not alone. Cancer can feel like a solo journey, but not when you're surrounded by such amazing people—people I never would have met had I not been diagnosed with cancer.

I'm not comfortable with the notion of "gifts of cancer" or even "finding the silver lining." The costs of cancer, both physically and emotionally, are a little too high to justify any bright sides. But because we all belong to the club, we may as well grab the perks when they come along.

For Rachel, who had stage-three breast cancer, the biggest gift was discovering the strength in herself. She's done things she never thought she could. "I had to rely more on myself for my happiness and my confidence," she says. "It took a lot of hard work, but I'm glad that I was able to turn this into a positive experience. Rather than something that's ruined my life, it's actually something that has made it better."

Jennifer, also a breast cancer survivor, learned appreciation. "All that's happened to you, really, is that the illusion of immortality has been removed," she says. "You start understanding that you're not going to live forever—and there's an incredible blessing to that," she says. "Because you don't waste time."

Joe, a survivor of non-Hodgkins lymphoma, learned perspective. "Cancer is probably the worst thing that ever happened to me, but it's also the best thing that ever happened to me," he explains, "because it gives me a unique perspective that some people will try their entire life to find." Thanks to cancer, Joe can truly appreciate every second. "You just never really know when your time's going to come, whether it's a car accident or cancer or whatever," says Joe. You have to embrace life and approach it as if each day is your last. I know that a lot of people use that as a cliché, but for me, that's a way of life."

"I absolutely, unequivocally changed as a person," says Joe. He used to be an extreme Type A personality. "But now I'm more relaxed and more cognizant of 'if it doesn't get done, it's not the end of the world.'" Now Joe takes a step back and looks at the big picture. "You've got your health or you've got your family or you've got whatever." That kind of perspective—focusing on what you do have—is what matters to Joe. Even when he loses someone, as he recently did, it urges Joe forward. "That aspect of it is really extremely difficult. But it also adds more fuel to the fire to give back, to do more."

For Khit, who has survived vulval cancer and melanoma, the gift was the people she met. Khit had a rough adolescence. To escape an arranged marriage and an oppressively traditional household, Khit ran away from home at age sixteen. The next few years were a jumble of high school and waiting tables, abusive relationships, and sleeping in her car. She felt alone, totally without support.

"When I had cancer and I found Imerman Angels [an organization that matches people touched by cancer with a mentor who'd had a similar experience], it was the first time where I was around people who actually could understand me." It was the first time Khit felt she belonged. "I feel like a lot of wonderful things come from traumatizing experiences. They kind of wake us up," she says. These days, Khit tries to live every day as though it were her last. "I find that that lets part of me let go of a lot of things that were causing bitterness and hate inside me."

Barbra, who had breast cancer, learned to ask for help. "It was hard for me to do that because I've been a giver my whole life—I don't like to ask for help," she explains. "I've always been the one in my family that's done for everybody." After her surgeries, though, Barbara couldn't do everything for herself. "It's very hard," she says. "But you learn. That is the good part of having cancer."

Some people found new careers: Ann realized that as much as she enjoyed fashion design, she was happier running a nutrition-focused nonprofit. Khit came to understand that medical school wasn't as meaningful to her as working in marketing and outreach for nonprofit organizations. Elissa moved from working in public health research to running a cancer survivorship services program.

I made strong and (hopefully lasting) friendships with people I probably wouldn't ever have met otherwise. I gained an appreciation for the little things in life, such as taking my son to try out for a Broadway show and touring colleges with my daughter.

Going through cancer allowed my children to show me their responsibility and compassion; after my double mastectomy, my sixteen-year-old daughter loaned me her computer and iPad while she was at sleepaway camp so that I could recuperate accompanied by Netflix, and my then-twelve-year-old son cooked and did the dishes, straightened up the living room, and did the wash at the Laundromat; I don't, however, recommend getting life-threatening diseases to find out whether your children are growing up to be empathetic and conscientious—though mine did pass the inadvertent test with flying colors.

Ultimately, though, probably the greatest lesson I have gained from cancer is a greater confidence in myself, a clearer sense of my own strength. Parenthood taught me to be flexible, and taught me how to educate and model. Divorce showed me that I could do the taxes and unclog the toilet (usually). Cancer taught me resilience and self-reliance, and gave me a belief in my own inner strength. If I can do cancer—diagnosis, treatment, and survivorship—then, damn it, I can do anything.

And so can you.

Acknowledgments

First, I would like to thank Delia Casa, Abigail Gehring, and the wonderful people at Skyhorse Publishing. This book would just be a twinkle in my eye if it were not for the people who brought it out into the world. I'd also like to mention Lee Thrash, who gave me the chance to start exploring some of these topics in print.

I'd also like to thank people who read the manuscript with careful eyes. Maya Hawkins, Michael Ishii, Julie Kahn, and Charles Salzberg and company provided important input on content and style. I am grateful for all the comments, though of course I take responsibility for any errors that remain. I'd also like to thank Percy Corcoran for immeasurable help with the index.

While I don't consider myself lucky to have had cancer, I have been extremely fortunate to have many wonderful people in my life who helped me throughout cancer treatment, recovery, and survivorship. I'm also lucky to have this forum to thank people, which reminds me: let me start out by apologizing in advance to anyone I fail to mention. Can we chalk it up to chemobrain?

PS 3 took me under its wing, and I am especially indebted, in alpha order, to Amie Schiendel, Andrea Frank, Charlotte DeWald, Charly Greene, Chin Koock and Joan Pierpoline, Claire Honig, Jennie Miller, Katherine Harrison, and Terry Spring-Robinson. Town and Village Synagogue was equally critical for me and my children, and I'd like to mention, in particular, Binyumen and Carol Schaechter, Cantor Shayna Postman, Efrat Pellet, Eva Heineman, Heli and

Jonathan David, Judith Keisman, Maude Keisman, Nikki and Ted Greenberg, Rabbi Larry Sebert, Roberta Schine, Shanee Epstein, and Sophie Riese. I'd also like to express my appreciation to colleagues Anne Fallucchi, Eileen McMorrow, Ingrid Edelman, and Lee Thrash. A special nod to folks in the cancer community, including Laura Mosiello, Mary Cahill, Stephen Malamud, Susan Boolbol, Wade Iwata, and the other folks at Beth Israel Medical Center, Gilda's Club NYC, CEW, and the Leukemia and Lymphoma Society. I'd like to extend a particular thank-you to Beth Holzback, Deni DeYonker, Delores Wilson, Mitria DiGiacomo, Wendy Sharff, Fran Weisberg, Percy Corcoran, Susan Blanchard, Haydee Lopez, and Ann Fry. And then there's Charles Salzberg and the crew at the JCC who were also wonderful, wonderful, wonderful.

Not to mention friends and relatives in New York, around the country, and in a few cases around the world, notably Ali and James Kaufman, Cindy Katz and Gili Chupak, Debbie Abbott, Debby Viveros, Donna Mather, Garo Green, Jane McAndrew, Jeanette Palmer, Jennifer Berman, Julie Kahn, Karen Eizman, Michelle Volpe, Olive Riffkin, Rachel Leibson, Rebecca Prigal, Roberta Levy-Schwartz, Scott Zachek, and Susan Silverman. A special thank-you to all those people—you know who you are, and there are more than I'd like to admit—who let me nap on your sofa while you fed and watered my children.

Most of all, a tremendously huge and enormous thank-you to Maya and Ari, who provided me—and continue to provide me—with enough chaos to keep me focused and enough joy to make it all worthwhile. I love you dearly, and, no, I don't have a favorite. (There, now I said it in print, so please stop asking.)

October 2013

Resources for Survivorship

General Cancer

American Cancer Society (ACS). Provides online support and public health education and funds cancer research. The Cancer Survivors Network offers member search, discussion boards, chat rooms, and private CSN e-mail. www.cancer.org/

American Institute for Cancer Research (AICR). Conducts research and has links to information on diet, nutrition, and cancer. Provides support groups, recipes, and tips for everyday changes that may lower risk for cancer recurrence and secondary cancers. www.aicr.org/

Association of Cancer Online Resources. Provides information and support to cancer patients and survivors and those who care for them through social networking, such as cancer-related Internet mailing lists and Web-based resources. www.acor.org/

CancerCare. Provides online and face-to-face support groups, phone and online education workshops, and online and print publications. www.cancercare.org/

CaringBridge. Allows patients and survivors to create a personal website, an online space to connect, share news, and receive support. www.caringbridge.org/

Gilda's Club. Offers free support groups, classes, and social events at clubhouses around the country. Also offers classes ranging from qigong to crocheting and from reiki to nutrition. www.gildasclubnyc.org/Membership/Programs.html

Imerman Angels. Pairs survivors with a "mentoring angel" who is of the same age and gender and has beaten the same type of cancer for information and support. www.imermanangels.org/

Journey Forward. Promotes use of survivorship care plans as a systematic approach to end-of-care treatment. The website offers a template care plan that can be individualized. http://journeyforward.org/

Livestrong Foundation. Provides support for people touched by cancer. Offers survivorship support groups, aid in developing a survivorship care plan, and information on exercise, nutrition, living with uncertainty, and other issues for survivors. www.livestrong.org/

Malecare. Offers in-person and online support for male cancer patients and survivors and their families. It is the first men's cancer survivor organization to focus on gay and bisexual men's survivorship. http://malecare.org/

MyLifeLine.org. Helps cancer patients and caregivers create free, customized websites. www.mylifeline.org/

National Cancer Institute (NCI) at the National Institutes of Health (NIH). Conducts and supports research, training, health information dissemination, and other programs with respect to the cause, diagnosis, prevention, and treatment of cancer, rehabilitation from cancer, and the continuing care of cancer patients and their families. www.cancer.gov/aboutnci

National Coalition for Cancer Survivorship (NCCS). Advocates for quality cancer care for all people touched by cancer and provides tools that empower people to advocate for themselves. Offers information on employment and health insurance issues. www.canceradvocacy.org/

Navigate Cancer Foundation. Provides one-on-one education, advocacy, and support to survivors and their friends and family members. Offers information on complementary treatments, financial support, clinical trials, support groups, and survivorship plans. www.navigatecancerfoundation.org/

Legal and Career

Cancer and Careers. Provides tools and information for employees with cancer, and offers publications, career coaching, support groups, and educational seminars focusing on career and legal issues. www.cancerandcareers.org

Cancer Legal Resource Center (CLRC). Provides information and education about cancer-related legal issues to the public. www.disabilityrightslegalcenter.org/cancer-legal-resource-center

Cancer Support Community. Provides support and information to people touched by cancer. www.cancersupportcommunity.org/default.aspx

Disability Rights Legal Center. Offers free legal service to people with disabilities, such as cancer. www.lls.edu/academics/centersprograms/disabilityrightslegalcenter/

Job Accommodation Network. Part of the U.S. Department of Labor, the organization provides free, expert, and confidential guidance on workplace accommodations and disability employment issues. www.askjan.org/

Tracy Fitzpatrick, coach and facilitator for life's transitions. Provides life and career coaching. www.tracyfitzpatrick.com/

Triage Cancer. Provides education and resources on issues of cancer survivorship. http://triagecancer.org/

Exercise and Nutrition

Cancer Climber Association. Offers grants for adventure trips for cancer survivors. http://cancerclimber.org/home.php

The Cancer Project. Provides research, education, and advocacy to promote cancer prevention and survival. Food for Life classes teach survivors and their families about healthy nutrition. http://pcrm.org/health/cancer-resources/

Cook for Your Life. Teaches healthy eating and cooking to cancer survivors. www.cfyl.org

Livestrong at the Y. Provides exercise training for cancer survivors. www.livestrong.org/What-We-Do/Our-Actions/Programs-Partnerships/LIVESTRONG-at-the-YMCA

Eastern and Alternative Modalities

American Massage Therapy Association. Provides referrals to qualified massage therapists. www.amtamassage.org/index.html

American Psychosocial Oncology Society (APOS). Provides referrals to local psychiatrists, psychologists, nurses, social workers, and counselors skilled in dealing with cancer-related distress. www.apos-society.org/survivors/helpline/helpline.aspx

American Reflexology Certification Board. Provides list of nationally certified reflexologists. http://arcb.net/cms/

American Society of Clinical Oncology (ASCO). Does advocacy, networking, and education aimed at psychosocial care of people with cancer, their families, and their caregivers. www.asco.org/

Center for Mindfulness in Medicine, Health Care, and Society. Provides listing of MBSR programs worldwide. www.umassmed. edu/cfm/index.aspx

International Center for Reiki Training. Provides access to Reiki masters who have agreed to abide by the organization's code of ethics and standards of practice. www.reikimembership.com/ MembershipListing.aspx

International Coach Federation. Provides access to professional coaches who have met stringent education and experience requirements, and have demonstrated mastery of the coaching competencies. www.coachfederation.org/need/landing.cfm?ItemNu mber=980&navItemNumber=569

National Cancer Center for Complementary and Alternative Medicine. Provides online information about the safety and efficacy of CAM treatments for cancer survivors. http://nccam.nih.gov/

National Certification Board for Therapeutic Massage & Bodywork. Provides referrals to board-certified massage therapists, organized by location. www.ncbtmb.org/

National Certification Commission for Acupuncture and Oriental Medicine (NCCAOM). Provides referrals to NCCAOM practitioners. www.nccaom.org/

Yoga Bear. Provides cancer patients and survivors with access to yoga in their communities and online. www.yogabear.org/

Yoga to the People. Provides low-cost yoga classes in New York City; Seattle; San Francisco; Berkeley, California; and Tempe, Arizona. http://yogatothepeople.com/

Young Survivors

Stupid Cancer. Offers resources, young adult conferences and social networking events, and a wide variety of outreach, awareness, and peer-connection programs. http://stupidcancer.org/

Surviving and Moving Forward. Provides direct financial assistance and in-person and online support to young adult cancer survivors. www.thesamfund.org/

Ulman Cancer Fund for Young Adults. Supports, educates, connects, and empowers young adult cancer survivors. http://ulmanfund.org/

Young Survival Coalition. The premier organization for young breast cancer patients and survivors; it offers information to plan care, manage health care, and access one-on-one support. www.youngsurvival.org/

Sexuality and Fertility

American Association of Sexuality Educators, Counselors and Therapists (AASECT). Provides referrals to sexuality educators around the country and around the world. www.aasect.org/default. aspx

American Society for Reproductive Medicine (ASRM). Provides information on reproductive medicine. www.asrm.org/ASRM_Publications_Overview/

Fertile Action. Helps women touched by cancer become mothers by offering peer-to-peer support, online support groups, and grants. www.fertileaction.org/

Fertile Hope. A Livestrong initiative, Fertile Hope provides reproductive information, support, funding, and hope to cancer patients and survivors whose medical treatments present the risk of infertility. http://fertilehope.org/

Gay and Lesbian Medical Association. Provides referrals to LGBT-friendly (lesbian, gay, bisexual, transgender) health-care providers. www.glma.org/index.cfm?fuseaction=Page.viewPage&pageId=939 &grandparentID=534&parentID=938&nodeID=1

International Society for the Study of Women's Sexual Health. Provides referrals to female sexual medical physicians. www.isswsh. org/resources/provider.aspx

MyOncoFertility.org. Offers patient education on issues of oncology and fertility. Provides survivor stories, written information, and videos for women as well as for men. www.myoncofertility.org/

Oncofertility Consortium. A national, interdisciplinary initiative designed to explore the reproductive future of cancer survivors. Provides information and resources. http://oncofertility. northwestern.edu/about-us

Save My Fertility. Online fertility preservation tool kit. www. savemyfertility.org/

Society for Assisted Reproductive Technologies (SART). Provides information on IVF facilities that are members of SART. www.sart. org/find_frm.html

Specific Cancers

Beverly Fund. Promotes lung cancer awareness and education, patient support, and early detection research. www.beverlyfund.org/

Bladder Cancer Advocacy Network. Provides information and support to the bladder cancer community, increases public awareness of bladder cancer, and advances research and funding for bladder cancer. www.bcan.org/

Kidney Cancer Association. Provides support and information for kidney cancer patients and survivors. www.kidneycancer.org/

Leukemia and Lymphoma Society. Provides information and support services for patients and survivors of leukemia, lymphoma, Hodgkin's disease, and myeloma. www.lls.org/

Liddy Shriver Sarcoma Initiative. Provides information about sarcoma and sarcoma research to individuals, families, communities, and medical teams around the world. www.sarcomahelp.org/

Living Beyond Breast Cancer. Offers programs and services to women affected by breast cancer, caregivers, and health-care providers. www.lbbc.org/

Lung Cancer Alliance. Provides support and advocacy for people living with or at risk for lung cancer. www.lungcanceralliance.org/

National Breast Cancer Foundation. Provides women with free mammograms, education, support, and early detection services. www.nationalbreastcancer.org/

National Lymphedema Network (NLN). Provides education and guidance to lymphedema patients, health-care professionals, and the general public. www.lymphnet.org/

Ovarian Cancer National Alliance. Advocates for women with ovarian cancer, conducts public education, and educates health-care professionals. www.ovariancancer.org/

Pancreatic Cancer Action Network. Provides reliable, personalized information. www.pancan.org/index.php

Sarcoma Alliance. Provides education, guidance, and support to sarcoma patients and survivors. http://sarcomaalliance.org/

SHARE Cancer Support. Offers support for women with breast cancer, metastatic breast cancer, and ovarian cancer. www.sharecancersupport.org/share-new/

Sharsheret. Offers information and support to young Jewish women facing breast and ovarian cancer and their families. www.sharsheret.org/

Susan G. Komen Breast Cancer Foundation. Provides funding for breast cancer research, education, advocacy, health services, and social support programs. http://ww5.komen.org/

Testicular Cancer Society. Offers support for patients, survivors, and caregivers. www.testicularcancersociety.org/

Us TOO Prostate Cancer Education and Support. Provides prostate cancer patients and their families with information, materials, and peer-to-peer support. www.ustoo.org/Default.asp

You Can Thrive. Offers free and low-cost preventative support services and long-term survivorship tools for breast cancer survivors. http://youcanthrive.org/

Body Mass Index Table

To use the table, find the appropriate height in the left-hand column labeled Height. Move across to a given weight (in pounds). The number at the top of the column is the BMI at that height and weight. Pounds have been rounded off. The chart is from the National Heart Lung and Blood Institute (NHLBI).

BMI	19	20	21	22	23	24	25	26	27	28	29	30	31	32	33	34	35
Height (inches)								Body Weight (pounds)									
58	91	96	100	105	110	115	119	124	129	134	138	143	148	153	158	162	167
59	94	99	104	109	114	119	124	128	133	138	143	148	153	158	163	168	173
60	97	102	107	112	118	123	128	133	138	143	148	153	158	163	168	174	179
61	100	106	111	116	122	127	132	137	143	148	153	158	164	169	174	180	185
62	104	109	115	120	126	131	136	142	147	153	158	164	169	175	180	186	191
63	107	113	118	124	130	135	141	146	152	158	163	169	175	180	186	191	197
64	110	116	122	128	134	140	145	151	157	163	169	174	180	186	192	197	204
65	114	120	126	132	138	144	150	156	162	168	174	180	186	192	198	204	210
66	118	124	130	136	142	148	155	161	167	173	179	186	192	198	204	210	216
67	121	127	134	140	146	153	159	166	172	178	185	191	198	204	211	217	223
68	125	131	138	144	151	158	164	171	177	184	190	197	203	210	216	223	230
69	128	135	142	149	155	162	169	176	182	189	196	203	209	216	223	230	236
70	132	139	146	153	160	167	174	181	188	195	202	209	216	222	229	236	243
71	136	143	150	157	165	172	179	186	193	200	208	215	222	229	236	243	250
72	140	147	154	162	169	177	184	191	199	206	213	221	228	235	242	250	258
73	144	151	159	166	174	182	189	197	204	212	219	227	235	242	250	257	265
74	148	155	163	171	179	186	194	202	210	218	225	233	241	249	256	264	272
75	152	160	168	176	184	192	200	208	216	224	232	240	248	256	264	272	279
76	156	164	172	180	189	197	205	213	221	230	238	246	254	263	271	279	287

Adapted from Clinical Guidelines on the Identification, Evaluation, and Treatment of Overweight and Obesity in Adults: The Evidence Report.

A Guide to Phytochemicals

Thousands of phytochemicals have been identified so far, and scientists have only begun to investigate their promise. This chart lists some of the phytochemicals now attracting serious scientific attention, identifies food sources, and outlines potential benefits.

Phytochemical(s)	Plant Source	Possible Benefits
Carotenoids (such as beta-carotene, lycopene, lutein, zeaxanthin)	Red, orange, and green fruits and vegetables, including broccoli, carrots, cooked tomatoes, leafy greens, sweet potatoes, winter squash, apricots, cantaloupe, oranges, and watermelon	May inhibit cancer cell growth, work as antioxidants, and improve immune response

(Continued)

Appendix III Table *(Continued)*

Phytochemical(s)	Plant Source	Possible Benefits
Flavonoids (such as anthocyanins and quercetin)	Apples, citrus fruits, onions, soybeans and soy products (tofu, soy milk, edamame, etc.), coffee, and tea	May inhibit inflammation and tumor growth; may aid immunity and boost production of detoxifying enzymes in the body
Indoles and glucosinolates (sulforaphane)	Cruciferous vegetables (broccoli, cabbage, collard greens, kale, cauliflower, and Brussels sprouts)	May induce detoxification of carcinogens, limit production of cancer-related hormones, block carcinogens, and prevent tumor growth
Inositol (phytic acid)	Bran from corn, oats, rice, rye and wheat, nuts, soybeans, and soy products, (tofu, soy milk, edamame, etc.)	May retard cell growth and work as antioxidant
Isoflavones (daidzein and genistein)	Soybeans and soy products (tofu, soy milk, edamame, etc.)	May inhibit tumor growth, limit production of cancer-related hormones, and generally work as antioxidant
Isothiocyanates	Cruciferous vegetables (broccoli, cabbage, collard greens, kale, cauliflower, and Brussels sprouts)	May induce detoxification of carcinogens, block tumor growth, and work as antioxidants

Phytochemical(s)	Plant Source	Possible Benefits
Polyphenols (such as ellagic acid and resveratrol)	Green tea, grapes, wine, berries, citrus fruits, apples, whole grains, and peanuts	May prevent cancer formation, prevent inflammation, and work as antioxidants
Terpenes (such as perillyl alcohol, limonene, and carnosol)	Cherries, citrus fruit peel, and rosemary	May protect cells from becoming cancerous, slow cancer cell growth, strengthen immune function, limit production of cancer-related hormones, fight viruses, and work as antioxidants

Index

A

AASECT (American Association of
　　Sexuality Educators, Counselors
　　and Therapists), 292
ACA (Affordable Care Act), 195–97
accommodation, reasonable, 187, 188,
　　190–94
accomplishments, 12, 171
ACOR (Association of Cancer Online
　　Resources), 287
ACS. *See* American Cancer Society
acupuncture, 241–42, 247–49
acupuncturists, 244
ADA (Americans with Disabilities Act)
　　confidentiality and, 186
　　interviews and, 159
　　job offers and, 184
　　preemptive action, 128
　　reasonable accommodation, 187, 190
　　state equivalents, 180
　　time off, 188, 189
aerobic exercise, 219
Affordable Care Act (ACA), 195–97
AICR (American Institute for Cancer
　　Research), 258–59
alcohol, 230
alive, feeling, 10–12, 170–71
alternative medicine. *See* complementary
　　modalities
American Association of Sexuality
　　Educators, Counselors and
　　Therapists (AASECT), 292
American Cancer Society (ACS)
　　on chat rooms, 273
　　on exercise trainers, 224
　　exercise guidelines, 217–18
　　on fertility, 96, 97–98
　　on guided imagery, 262
　　Hope Lodge, 15
　　on massage, 266–67

on moxa, 248–49
on recurrence fears, 25
on Reiki, 263
on signs of recurrence, 33–34
on support groups, 273
website, 287
on weight, 216, 234–35
on yoga, 268–69
American College of Sports Medicine,
　　224
American Institute for Cancer Research
　　(AICR)
　　on grilling, 233–34
　　on nutrition, 229–231
　　on phytochemicals, 231–32
　　on soy, 232–33
　　on supplements, 258–59
　　on underweight, 235
　　website, 287
American Massage Therapy Association
　　(AMTA), 290
American Psychosocial Oncology Society
　　(APOS), 275, 290
American Reflexology Certification
　　Board, 290
American Society for Reproductive
　　Medicine (ASRM), 93, 99, 107,
　　292
American Society of Clinical Oncology
　　(ASCO), 203, 209, 291
Americans with Disabilities Act. *See* ADA
AMTA (American Massage Therapy
　　Association), 290
analyzing, 12–14
antibiotics, 236
anxiety. *See also* depression; fear
　　appointments and, 29–30, 208
　　career changes, 174–76
　　complementary modalities and, 257
　　exercise and, 225

job changes, 150
post-treatment, 46–48
sexual problems and, 69, 81
treatments, 61–62
triggers, 43
volunteering and, 17
work, returning to, 124–25
APOS (American Psychosocial Oncology Society), 275, 290
appointments, 29–30, 208
arousal, 70
ASCO (American Society of Clinical Oncology), 203, 209, 291
Asian medicine. *See* East Asian medicine
ASRM (American Society for Reproductive Medicine), 93, 99, 107, 292
Association of Cancer Online Resources (ACOR), 287
astragalus, 251
Atlantic Reproductive Center, 102
attitude, 13–14, 55–58, 170
Audrey, 270

B
Bantug, Elissa
appointment anxiety, 29
on caregivers, 32–33
job change, 143–44
mastectomy, 37
on people's responses, 117
on recovery, 30–31
on recurrence fear, 26–27, 28
on recurrence fears, 24–25, 34–35
on sexual problems, 65–66, 68–69, 75
on support groups, 32
triggers, 30
on volunteering, 14, 17
on wellness, 200
on worrying, 37
barbequing, 233–34
Barbra, 14–15, 111, 177–78, 282–83
baths, 73
BCAN (Bladder Cancer Advocacy Network), 293
behavior modification therapy, 275
Believing in Magic (Vyse), 51
Bender, Alice, 258–59
Beth, 15, 255–56
Beverly Fund, 293
Bikram yoga, 269
bilateral mastectomy, 37, 255

birth control, 108–9
birth problems, 96, 109, 110
bladder cancer, 97
Bladder Cancer Advocacy Network (BCAN), 293
blogging, 155, 156, 264–65
blood cancers, 4, 67
BMI (Body Mass Index), 217, 234, 297–98
body image, 70–74
Body Mass Index (BMI), 217, 234, 297–98
bosses. *See* supervisors
Boston Globe, 57
brain cancer, 14, 42, 67, 75, 203
BRCA testing, 101
breast cancer,
antibiotics and, 236
birth control and, 108–9
body image and, 70–71, 73
coping styles and, 59-60
dating and, 82–83, 86
exercise and, 214–15, 219, 220
fertility and, 100, 102, 103
hair loss and, 50
health care, primary and, 209
herbal therapy, 251
Hodgkin's survivors and, 203
John's Hopkins Survivorship Program, 144
lymphedema and, 125
qigong and, 252
relationships and, 111, 118
sexual problems and, 65, 67, 68, 76
soy and, 232–33
Tamoxifen and, 207
unemployment and, 121
weight and, 215, 216–17, 234
work, returning to, 135–6
breast reconstruction, 73, 74, 255
breast removal, 36–37, 73, 255
breastfeeding, 110

C
CAM (complementary and alternative medicine). *See* complementary modalities
cancer
bladder, 97
brain, 14, 42, 67, 75, 203
breast, *see* breast cancer
children and, 105

in East Asian medicine, 245–46
emotional challenges, 46–48
endometrial, 121, 125, 168
hemotological, 4, 67
Hodgkin's lymphoma, 27, 89, 112, 203, 211
job loss and, 177–79
kidney, 163, 165, 216
lessons from, 281–83
metaphor for evil, 25
non-Hodgkin's lymphoma, 15, 89, 224, 281
nutrition and, 229–231
obesity and, 216–17, 234–35
ovarian, 68, 90–91, 121, 125, 168–69
prostate, *see* prostate cancer
rates, x–xi
second primary, 35–37
sexual problems and, 66–67
signs of, 33–34
soy and, 232–33
stigma, 25
vulval, 82, 267, 282
Cancer and Careers
  on disclosure, 134, 182
  on interviews, 159
  on meaningful work, 172
  on resumes, 154
  on returning to work, 139–140
  website, 289
  on work-life balance, 133
Cancer Climber Association, 290
Cancer Legal Resource Center (CLRC), 289
Cancer Project, 290
Cancer Support Community, 289
CancerCare, 287
CancerCare Manitoba, 66, 77
career changes. *See also* jobs; work
  Ann's story, 163–67
  anxiety, 174–76
  examples, 283
  exploring, 173–74
  Khit's story, 167–68
  priorities and, 169–173
  short-term, 168–69
  volunteering and, 17
career choices, 121
CareerBuilder, 156
caregivers, 32–33
carotenoids, 299
CaringBridge, 155, 288

CDC (Centers for Disease Control and Prevention), 106, 256
Center for Mindfulness in Medicine, Health Care, and Society, 291
Centers for Disease Control and Prevention (CDC), 106, 256
chat rooms, 15, 273
"chemobrain," 125
"chemo-pause," 96, 215
chemotherapy, 96, 97–98, 103, 215–16
chi. *See* qi
children, 105
cholesterol, 230
Chris, 178–79
clothing, 160, 161
CLRC (Cancer Legal Resource Center), 289
cognitive therapy, 275
Collins, Karen, 232
colorectal cancer, 209
Columbia University, 167
communication, 75, 77, 130–31, 135, 194
Community Supported Agriculture (CSA), 227–28, 237
commuting, 128
complementary modalities. *See also* East Asian medicine
  explained, 256–58
  guided imagery, 261–62
  journaling, 263–65
  massage, 265–67
  meditation, 260–61
  probiotics, 259
  reflexology, 269–270
  Reiki, 262–63
  resources, 290–91
  support groups, 270–74
  therapy, 274–77
  vitamin supplements, 258–59
  yoga, 267–69
conditioning, 44
confidence, 19, 83–84, 152
confidentiality, 187
Connecticut College, 51, 200
consulting, 153
contingency planning, 136–37
control, 12–13, 99, 199–200
Cook For Your Life, 166, 290
coping styles. *See also* attitude, 58–59, 59–61
Copland, Susannah, 102

corn, 236
counseling, *see* therapy
couples therapy, 275
critics, internal. *See also* "gremlins,"
    19–21
cryopreservation. *See* freezing
CSA (Community Supported Agriculture),
    227–28, 237
curcuma, 251

D
dairy products, 229, 231, 236, 259
"daisy chain," 113–14
Dana Farber Cancer Institute, 15, 47,
    177, 214
dating, 72, 75–76, 82–86
"defensive pessimism," 57
Deni, 227–29
denial, 5
Department of Health and Human
    Services, 196
Department of Labor, 183, 185, 187–88,
    189, 190
depression. *See also* anxiety, 41, 46–48,
    61–62, 69, 257
desire, sexual, 70
desks, 138
Destin, Daniel, 214, 219, 222–23, 224
diet. *See* nutrition
dilators, 79
disability, 126, 159, 184–96, 204
Disability Rights Legal Center, 189, 190,
    195, 289
disclosure
    current employers, 186
    explained, 181–82
    interviewing and, 183–86
    Julie's story, 130
    medical leave and, 182–83
    process, 186–87
    resumes and, 153
discrimination, employment, 194–95
divorce, 13
Donna
    on relationships, 117, 117–18
    on work relationships, 129–130, 133,
        134
    on working, 123–24, 127–29
    on work-life balance, 135
double mastectomy, 36–37, 255
Doyle, Colleen, 218, 219, 221–22, 225

E
E. coli, 236
Early Retiree Reinsurance Program
    (ERRP), 197
East Asian medicine. *See also*
    complementary modalities
    acupuncture, 247–49
    cancer according to, 245–46
    explained, 239–243
    herbal therapy, 250–52
    human body in, 243–44
    moxibustion, 248–49
    nutrition, 249–250
    physical manipulation, 253
    qigong, 252–53
    resources, 290–91
eating. *See* nutrition
ED (erectile dysfunction), 77
education, 139–140
EEOC (Equal Employment Opportunity
    Commission), 184, 186, 187
eggs, 101–2, 106–7
Ehrenreich, Barbara, 57
Elissa. *See* Bantug, Elissa
embryos, 99–101
Emory University, 47
emotional challenges, 46–48, 68, 246
employment. *See* career changes; jobs;
    work
end of life, 18
endometrial cancer, 121, 125, 168
engagement, 10–12, 170–71, 173
ephedra, 251
Equal Employment Opportunity
    Commission (EEOC), 184, 186,
    187
erectile dysfunction (ED), 77
ergonomics, 137–39, 140
ERRP (Early Retiree Reinsurance
    Program), 197
Evanson, Annalise, 200, 262–63, 269,
    276
exercise
    ACS guidelines, 217–18
    benefits, 225
    cancer and, 214–15
    emotional health and, 61
    peaceful, 224–25
    recommendations, 221–22
    recurrence and, 128
    resources, 290
    sexual health and, 87

timing, 221–22
Tito's story, 211–13
trainers, 223–24
Yael's story, 213–14

F
Facebook, 155, 156, 158
faith, 17–19, 212
Family Medical Leave Act (FMLA), 123,
    180, 183, 188–190
FDA (Food and Drug Administration),
    251, 259
fear. *See also* anxiety
    of appointments, 29–30, 208
    of career changes, 174–76
    of job changes, 150
    of places, 43–45
    of recurrence, 24–25, 26–28, 261
Fertile Action, 106, 109, 292
Fertile Hope, 292–93
fertility
    children and, 105
    drugs, 99, 107
    in men, 97–98
    post-treatment, 105–7
    preparation, 98–99
    preserving, 99–105
    resources, 292
    screening, 106, 107
    stories, 89–95
    in women, 95–97
Fitzpatrick, Tracy
on accomplishments, 12
    cancer diagnosis, 6–8
    on career changes, 169–171, 173–74,
        174–76
    on engagement, 10
    on gratitude, 42
    on inner critics, 20, 174–76
    on job changes, 149–150
    on mortality, 8–9
    on support groups, 32
    values, 11–12
    on volunteering, 17
    website, 290
flavonoids, 300
Flowerpot, Florence, 18
FMLA (Family Medical Leave Act), 123,
    180, 183, 188–190
food. *See* nutrition
Food and Drug Administration (FDA),
    251, 259

freezing
    eggs, 101–2
    embryos, 99–101
    ovarian tissue, 102–3
    sperm, 104
friends, 114–15, 119
From Cancer Patient to Cancer Survivor,
    203
fruit, 231, 258
fulfillment, 13

G
Gay and Lesbian Medical Association
    (GLMA), 293
Genentech, 209
genetic testing, 101
genetically modified organisms (GMOs),
    235–37
Genetics and IVF Institute, 98, 99
Gibson-Moore, Hannah H., 19, 264
Gilda's Club, 270–72, 288
giving back, 14–17
GLMA (Gay and Lesbian Medical
    Association), 293
glucosinolates, 300
GMOs (genetically modified organisms),
    235–37
Goldfarb, Shari, 71, 72, 74–75, 79
Google, 27, 155, 158
grains, 230, 231
gratitude, 144, 268
Greenstein, Mindy
    on cancer as metaphor, 25
    on coping styles, 48, 57, 58–59, 59–60
    on depression, 41–42
    on relationships, 113–15, 115–16
    on superstition, 50, 53
    on therapy, 275
    on volunteering, 17
"gremlins," 20–21, 174–76, 275
grieving, 118
grilling, 233–34
group therapy, 275
growth hormones, 236
guided imagery, 261–62
Guidelines on Nutrition and Physical
    Activity for Cancer Prevention,
    218
guilt, 15
Gynecologic Education and Awareness
    Act, 169

H

hair loss, 50, 83, 112, 132, 212
Haring, Lauren, 99, 101
Hatha yoga, 268
HCAs (hetero-cyclic amines), 233, 234
Health and Human Services, 196
health insurance, 11, 195–97
hemotological cancer, 4, 67
herbal therapy, 250–52
herbalists, 244
hetero-cyclic amines (HCAs), 233, 234
Hodgkin's lymphoma, 27, 89, 112, 203, 211
Hope Lodge, 15
hormone therapy, 68
HR (human resources), 133–34, 187
hysterectomy, 104

I

I Don't Know What I Want. (Jansen), 124
ICSI (intracytoplasmic sperm injection), 104
Ilana, 90–95
Imerman Angels, 15, 16–17, 82, 167–68, 282, 288
impotence, 75–77
in vitro fertilization (IVF), 100–101, 104, 107
incontinence, 80–81
indoles, 300
infections, 125–26
infertility. *See* fertility
inositol, 300
Institute for Traditional Medicine, 251
Institute of Medicine (IOM), x, 126, 203, 204–6, 208–9
Institute of Traditional Medicine, 247
integrated medicine. *See* complementary modalities
intentions, 13–14
International Center for Reiki Training, 263, 291
International Coach Federation, 291
International Society for the Study of Women's Sexual Health (ISSWSH), 293
interviewing, 159–161, 183–86
interviews, informational, 173–74
intracytoplasmic sperm injection (ICSI), 104
IOM (Institute of Medicine), x, 126, 203, 204–6, 208–9

Ishii, Michael
    on acupuncture, 240–42, 247
    on cancer, 243
    on herbal therapy, 250
    on nutrition, 249
    on physical manipulation, 253
    on qi, 243–44, 245, 246
isoflavones, 232–33, 300
isothiocyanates, 300
ISSWSH (International Society for the Study of Women's Sexual Health), 293
IVF (in vitro fertilization), 100–101, 104, 107

J

JAN (Job Accommodation Network), 190–94, 289
Jansen, Julie
    on career changes, 124–25
    on contingency planning, 136
    on disclosure, 130–31, 133–34
    on job searching, 151, 152
    on resumes, 153
    on work relationships, 132
    on work-life balance, 135
Jennifer, 281
Joanna's Law, 169
Job Accommodation Network (JAN), 190–94, 289
Job Searching with Social Media for Dummies (Waldman), 157
jobs. *See also* career changes; work
    annoyance with, 11–12
    changing, 51–52, 143–44, 146, 150–51
    interviewing, 159–161
    loss, 177–79
    resumes, 152–54
    satisfaction, 149
    search, 145–150, 151–52
    social media and, 155–58
Joe, 15–16, 89–90, 224–25, 281–82
Johns Hopkins Cancer Survivorship Programs, 14, 25, 45, 143–44, 273
Johns Hopkins Hospital, 8, 13
Johns Hopkins School of Medicine, 208
journaling, 263–65
Journey Forward, 209, 288
Julie, 130

K

Kabat-Zinn, John, 260
karate, 18
Katz, Anne, 66–67, 69–70, 72, 77, 109
Kegel exercises, 80–81
Khit, 16–17, 82, 167–68, 267–68, 282
kidney cancer, 163, 165, 216
Kidney Cancer Association, 294
Kojima, Ailin
   on emotional problems, 239–240
   on herbal therapy, 252
   on nutrition, 249
   on physical manipulation, 253
   on qi, 244, 245
   on Qigong, 252–53
Komen Foundation, 16, 86, 143, 259, 295
Kripalu Center for Yoga and Health, 18
Krychman, Michael, 109
Kups, Kathy-Ellen, 265

L

Lake Tahoe, 15, 224
Larson, Margot, 145–49, 159, 160
LBBC (Living Beyond Breast Cancer), 16, 86, 108–9, 294
legal issues
   accommodation, 190–94
   disclosure, 181–88
   discrimination, 194–95
   health insurance, 195–97
   researching, 180–81
   resources, 289–290
   time off, 188–190
Leukemia and Lymphoma Society (LLS), 16, 224, 294
libido, 68–69
Liddy Shriver Sarcoma Initiative, 294
life choices, 12–14
life coach, 145–46, 172–73
life-work balance, 121, 122, 133, 134–36, 145
lifting, 138
lighting, 74
Ligibel, Jennifer, 214–15, 221, 222
Lincoln, Stephen R.
   on fertility, 98, 104, 105, 106
   on freezing eggs, 101–2
   on freezing embryos, 99–100, 101
   on timing, 108
Lindsey, 199–200, 216
LinkedIn, 156, 157–58

Livestrong at the Y, 290
Livestrong Foundation
   on depression, 46
   Elissa and, 143
   exercise trainers, 224
   Joe and, 15
   on journaling, 264
   on parabens, 78
   on spirituality, 19
   website, 288
Living Beyond Breast Cancer (LBBC), 16, 86, 108–9, 294
LLS (Leukemia and Lymphoma Society), 16, 224, 294
low sperm count, 97, 104, 105, 107, 110
lubricants, 78
Lung Cancer Alliance, 294
lymphedema, 125
lymphoma
   Hodgkin's, 27, 89, 112, 203, 211
   non-Hodgkin's, 15, 89, 224, 281

M

magical thinking, 54
make-up, 160–61
Malecare, 274, 288
managers. *See* supervisors
manipulation, physical. *See* physical manipulation
marinating, 234
marriage, 11
mastectomy, 36–37, 73, 255
masturbation, 74, 104
Matasar, Matthew J., 202–3, 204, 205, 209
Matthew. *See* Zachary, Matthew
Mayo Clinic, 19, 56
MBSR (mindfulness-based stress reduction), 260–61
McFerrin, Bobby, 56
MD Anderson Cancer Center
   on body image, 71
   on emotional problems, 46
   on fertility, 95, 97, 103
   on lubricants, 78
   on qigong, 252
   on sex after cancer, 81
   on sexual problems, 67
   on vaginal atrophy, 79
meaning, 10–12, 17, 19, 170, 171–72
meat, 229, 231, 233–34, 236–37
medical leave, 183

Medicare, xi
medication, 68, 77
meditation, 18, 260–61
Memorial Sloan-Kettering Cancer Center, 68, 71, 202
memory loss, 13, 125
menopause, 96, 215–16
menstruation, 96–97, 99, 103, 106
Merschdorf, Jennifer, 215, 216, 220–21
milk, 229, 231, 236
milk products, 231, 259
milkshakes, 235
Miller, Andrew, 47
millettia, 251
mind and body medicine
    guided imagery, 261–62
    journaling, 263–65
    meditation, 260–61
    Reiki, 262–63
mindfulness-based stress reduction (MBSR), 260–61
Mindy. *See* Greenstein, Mindy
Miriam, 11
Morales, Joanna, 180, 183, 188, 189, 194–95
Moran, John, 122
mortality, xi, 8–9, 114
mourning, 118
Movember, 15
moxibustion, 248
MyLifeLine.org, 288
MyOncoFertility.org, 293

N
National Breast Cancer Foundation, 294
National Cancer Center for Complementary and Alternative Medicine, 291
National Cancer Institute (NCI), 15, 29, 66, 266, 288
National Center for Complementary and Alternative Medicine (NCCAM), 247, 251–52, 257–58, 266, 269
National Certification Board for Therapeutic Massage & Bodywork, 291
National Certification Commission for Acupuncture and Oriental Medicine (NCCAOM), 244, 248, 291
National Coalition for Cancer Survivorship (NCCS), 209, 289

National Heart Lung and Blood Institute (NHLBI), 297
National Institutes of Health (NIH), 143, 167, 201, 217, 234
National Lymphedema Network (NLN), 294
Navigate Cancer Foundation, 289
NCCAM (National Center for Complementary and Alternative Medicine), 247, 251–52, 257–58, 266, 269
NCCAOM (National Certification Commission for Acupuncture and Oriental Medicine), 244, 248, 291
NCCS (National Coalition for Cancer Survivorship), 209, 289
NCI (National Cancer Institute), 15, 29, 66, 266, 288
negetivity, 132–33
Nellis, Rebecca, 133–34, 182, 185, 187
networking, 173–74
neuropathy, 125, 223
Newton-Wellesley Hospital, 214, 222–23
NHLBI (National Heart Lung and Blood Institute), 297
NIH (National Institutes of Health), 143, 167, 201, 217, 234
nitrates, 236
NLN (National Lymphedema Network), 294
Non-GMO Project, 235
non-Hodgkin's lymphoma, 15, 89, 224, 281
Noogieland, 270–72
normalcy, 135
nurses, 138
nutrition
    AICR recommendations, 229–231
    East Asian medicine, 240, 249–252
    emotional health and, 61
    phytochemicals, 231–32, 299–301
    probiotics, 259
    resources, 290
    sexual health and, 87
    soy, 232–33
    vitamin supplements, 258–59

O
obesity, 216–17, 234–35
obsessive-compulsive disorder (OCD), 54–55

Occupational Safety and Health
    Administration (OSHA), 137–39
OCD (obsessive-compulsive disorder),
    54–55
OCNA (Ovarian Cancer National
    Alliance), 168–69, 171, 294
office politics, 131–32
Ogden, Anne, 163–67
oils, 229
oldenlandia, 251
OncoFertility Consortium, 107, 293
oncologists, 208
One Voice Against Cancer, 16
online reputation, 155–58
oocytes, 106
optimism, 55–58, 58–59, 61, 148, 212
organic food, 227–28, 235–37
organophosphate, 236
orgasm, 81
OSHA (Occupational Safety and Health
    Administration), 137–39
ostomy, 80
ova, 101–2, 106–7
ovarian cancer, 68, 90–91, 121, 125,
    168–69
Ovarian Cancer National Alliance
    (OCNA), 168–69, 171, 294
ovarian tissue, 102–3
oyster shell, 251

P
Pacific College of Oriental Medicine, 249,
    250
PAHs (polycyclic aromatic
    hydrocarbons), 233, 234
Pancreatic Cancer Action Network, 294
parabens, 78
Park Slope Food Co-op, 227
Pascal, Blaise, 53
"paying forward," 14–17
peace, 18, 224–25
Peale, Norman Vincent, 56
Pennsylvania State University, 122
periods, 96–97, 99, 103, 106
personal trainers, 223–24
personal values, 146–47
perspective, 37
pessimism. See also realism, 57
PET (positron emission tomography)
    scan, xii, 24, 29
physical manipulation
    East Asian medicine, 253

massage, 265–67
    reflexology, 269–270
    yoga, 267–69
physical therapy, 75, 79
phytochemicals, 231–32, 299–301
Pilates, 213–14
pivoting, 158
politics, office, 131–32
polycyclic aromatic hydrocarbons
    (PAHs), 233, 234
polyphenols, 301
port, x, 43
positive thinking, 55–58, 58–59, 61, 148,
    212
positron emission tomography (PET)
    scan, xii, 24, 29
poultry, 228, 229, 231, 233–34, 236
Power of Positive Thinking (Peale), 56
pre-existing conditions, 195–96
pregnancy. See also fertility, 98, 108–10
President's Cancer Panel, 203
priorities, 10–12, 145, 148–49
privacy, 187
probiotics, 259
processed foods, 230, 249
processed meats, 229, 233, 236, 237
prostate cancer
    exercise and, 214
    fertility and, 97
    health care, primary and, 209
    sexual problems and, 67, 68, 76
    weight and, 217, 234
protein, 229, 231
PS 3, ix–x
psycho-oncology, 275
psychosocial support
    support groups, 270–74
    therapy, 274–77
psychotherapy. See therapy
Pure Romance, 79
pyscho-oncologists, 275

Q
qi, 243–44, 245, 247, 252–53
qigong, 252–53

R
Rachel, 16, 82–83, 85–86, 103, 118–19,
    281
radiation, 105
rBGH, 236
Reach for Recovery, 14

realism, 57, 58–59, 61
reasonable accommodation, 187, 188, 190–94
reconstruction, breast, 73, 74, 255
recovery, 30–31
recurrence
    exercise and, 128, 214–15
    fear of, 24–25, 26–28, 261
    obesity and, 216–17
    second primary vs., 36–37
    signs of, 33–35
    soy and, 232–33
reflexology, 269–270
Reiki, 262–63
rejection, 174
relationships
    cancer and, 11, 111–15, 117–120
    coping, 115–17
    disclosure and, 181–82
    journaling and, 263
    work, 129–133, 133–34
religion, 17–19, 212
reputation, online, 155–58
resumes, 152–54
Retholz, Elaine, 260
Robert Half, 132
Roberta, 17–19
Rochelle, 29–30, 51–52, 150–51

S
Salmonella, 236
Sarcoma Alliance, 294
SART (Society for Assisted Reproductive Technologies), 293
saturated fatty acids, 230
Save My Fertility, 293
scarring, 70–71, 73
seafood, 229
second primary cancer, 35–37
self-blame, 54
self-delusion, 56–57
sexual problems
    cancer and, 66–67
    causes, 68–69
    exercise and, 225
    impotence, 75–77
    orgasm, 81
    painful sex, 77–78
    partners and, 69–70, 74–75
    resources, 292
    sex drive, 68–69
    wellness and, 87

SHARE Cancer Support, 295
Sharsheret, 295
Sherry, 125–26, 168–69, 171
Shipley Fitness Center, 214, 222–23
Shockney, Lillie, 8–9, 13, 45–46, 273
Shrover, Leslie, 67, 71, 77, 78, 80, 81
silver linings, 281–83
smoothies, 235
snacks, 229–230
Snyder, Claire, 208
social media, 155–58
Society for Assisted Reproductive Technologies (SART), 293
sodium, 230
sophora root, 251
Southern California Center for Sexual Health, 109
soy, 232–33
sperm, 104, 105, 107, 110
spirituality, 17–19, 212
St. John's wort, 258
strength training, 219
strengths, 147–48
stigma, 25
stress,
    exercise and, 225
    pregnancy and, 109
    sexual problems and, 69, 81
Stupid Cancer, 14, 274, 292
sugar, 230
superstition, 48–55, 113–14, 150
supervisors, 133–34, 149, 187
supplements, 258–59
support groups, 270–74
    career changes, 173
    post-treatment, 31–32
    work, returning to, 137
Surviving and Moving Forward, 292
survivors
    emotional challenges, 46–48
    Medicare and, xi
    oncologist relationship, 208
survivor's guilt, 15
survivorship care plans, 202–7, 209–10
Susan G. Komen Foundation, 16, 86, 143, 259, 295

T
Tamoxifen, 92, 94, 215, 228
Taylor, Shelley E., 200
TCM (traditional Chinese medicine), 242, 249

Teacher in the House (Jeremy), 280
Team in Training, 15, 224
terpenes, 301
testicular cancer, 97
Testicular Cancer Society, 295
testicular tissue, 105
Thai massage, 253
therapists, 274–75
therapy
    body image, 72
    individual, 274–77,
    physical, 75, 79
    sexual, 70, 75, 87
    work and, 137
time, 30–31, 72
time off, 188–190
timing pregnancy, 98, 108
Tito, 27, 89, 112, 211–13
tobacco, 230
Tour de Pink, 220–21
Tracy. *See* Fitzpatrick, Tracy
traditional Chinese medicine (TCM), 242, 249
trainers, personal, 223–24
trans fatty acid, 230
treatment
    fertility and, 93, 103–4, 105
    history, 204–5
    long-term effects, 206
    sexual problems and, 66–67
    transitioning, 202–3
    work and, 180–81
Triage Cancer, 180, 290
triggers, 30, 43–44
Tui-Na, 253
Twitter, 156, 158

U
UCLA (University of California Los Angeles), 200, 209
Ulman Cancer Fund for Young Adults, 292
underweight, 235
unemployment. *See also* work, 121
University of California Los Angeles (UCLA), 200, 209
University of Manitoba, 66, 77
University of Massachusetts, 260
University of Texas, 67
U.S. Department of Health and Human Services, 196

U.S. Department of Labor, 183, 185, 187–88, 189, 190
Us TOO, 295
uterus, 104

V
vaginal atrophy, 79
vaginal moisturizers, 79
values, 10–12, 146–47
vegetables, 229, 231, 234, 258
Viagra, 69
visualization, 11–12, 261–62
vitamin supplements, 258–59
volunteering, 14–17
vulval cancer, 82, 267, 282
Vyse, Stuart, 51, 52, 53–54, 55, 200

W
Waldman, Joshua, 157–58
war metaphors, 25
warning signs
    emotional, 47–48
    recurrence, 33–34
weight, 160, 215–17, 216–17, 234–35
WellPoint, Inc., 209
whole grains, 231
wig, 50-51
work. *See also* career changes; jobs
    cancer and, 180–81
    changes at, 126–29
    contingency plans, 136–37
    discrimination, 194–95
    ergonomics, 137–39
    meaningful, 170–73
    medical leave, 183
    preparing for, 136–37
    relationships, 129–133, 133–34
    returning to, 124–26, 136–37, 139–140
    supervisors, 133–34, 149, 187
    time off, 188–190
    transitioning, 139–140
    unemployment, 121
workaholics, 45–46
work-life balance, 121, 122, 133, 134–36, 145
worrying, 37–38

Y
Yael, 70–71, 213–14
yeast infections, 79
YMCA, 224, 290

yoga, 18, 253, 267–69
Yoga Bear, 291
Yoga to the People, 291
Yosemite, 11–12
You Can Thrive, 15, 256, 295
Young Survival Coalition (YSC), 216,
        220–21, 274, 292
yuan qi, 245

Z
Zachary, Matthew, 14, 42–43, 75–76,
        202
zedoria, 251
Zumba, 213–14

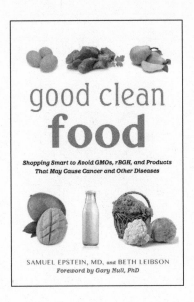

Good Clean Food

Shopping Smart to Avoid GMOs, rBGH, and Products That May Cause Cancer and Other Diseases

by Samuel Epstein, MD, and Beth Leibson

Foreword by Gary Null, PhD

Did you know that American milk and meat are banned in Europe because of the health risks they pose? Or that one in three items on supermarket shelves contains genetically modified ingredients? How about that forty pesticides in use today have been linked to certain types of cancer?

Between GMOs, hormones, and pesticides, it sometimes feels like our food has become so artificial that shopping smart is impossible. How can we know for sure that the food we buy isn't putting us at risk? If you've got questions, this practical, positive guide has answers. In it, leading public health advocate Samuel Epstein, MD, and coauthor Beth Leibson provide all of the information you need to make the best food choices for you and your family—in language you don't need a PhD in biology to understand.

$24.95 Hardcover • ISBN 978-1-61608-821-7

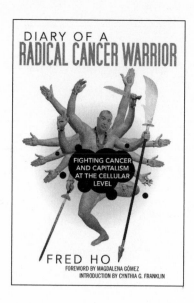

Diary of a Radical Cancer Warrior
Fighting Cancer and Capitalism at the Cellular Level
by Fred Ho
Foreword by Magdalena Gómez
Introduction by Cynthia G. Franklin

When American saxophonist and social activist Fred Ho was diagnosed with stage 3B colorectal cancer in 2006 he underwent immediate surgery to remove the tumor and began preparing for chemotherapy. Within days his friends mobilized to arrange grocery deliveries, transport, companionship, and housekeeping duties—they called themselves "Warriors for Fred."

Fred chose to write his astonishing cancer memoir as a diary, acknowledging that all the greatest warriors from Sun Tzu to swordsman Musasashi to Bruce Lee wrote daily diaries because warfare against a most formidable enemy will be won, ultimately, on the philosophical level. With incredibly detailed entries Fred talks frankly about his battle—his meticulous research, his various treatments, his successes, and his failures.

Above all, we learn what it means to truly live in the present—through Fred's unflinching description of the effects of colon cancer—and about his search not just for "a cure" in a medical sense, but for true healing. For Fred, this includes understanding the way of the warrior—one who fights for beauty, justice, health, equity, and sustainability.

$24.95 Hardcover • ISBN 978-1-61608-378-6

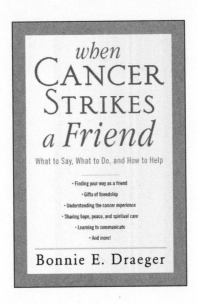

When Cancer Strikes a Friend

What to Say, What to Do, and How to Help

by Bonnie E. Draeger

Wondering what to say, how to help, and/or what to know about your friend with cancer? Now, for the first time, your questions will be answered in this supportive and instructional guide on how to be there for your loved one in his or her time of need. *When Cancer Strikes a Friend* is a prescriptive, step-by-step guide with menus of tried-and-true responses, bulleted examples, detailed sidebars, and sound advice from cancer professionals.

In Bonnie Draeger's debut book, professionals provide authoritative treatments of topics, including post-treatment; when friends live alone; pediatric and teen cancer issues; talking to children about cancer; and food, teamwork, and more. Featuring more than forty expert contributions, *When Cancer Strikes a Friend* is the essential guide for friends and colleagues who truly want to help their friends and family—acting as caregivers, listeners, and supporters—fight a winning battle against the Big C.

$14.95 Paperback • ISBN 978-1-62087-214-7